3251 Riverport Lane
St. Louis, Missouri 63043

Workbook for Pharmacology for Pharmacy Technicians 2 ed.   ISBN: 978-0-323-08498-7

Notices

Knowledge and best practice in this field are constantly changing. As new research and experience broaden our understanding, changes in research methods, professional practices, or medical treatment may become necessary.

Practitioners and researchers must always rely on their own experience and knowledge in evaluating and using any information, methods, compounds, or experiments described herein. In using such information or methods they should be mindful of their own safety and the safety of others, including parties for whom they have a professional responsibility.

With respect to any drug or pharmaceutical products identified, readers are advised to check the most current information provided (i) on procedures featured or (ii) by the manufacturer of each product to be administered, to verify the recommended dose or formula, the method and duration of administration, and contraindications. It is the responsibility of practitioners, relying on their own experience and knowledge of their patients, to make diagnoses, to determine dosages and the best treatment for each individual patient, and to take all appropriate safety precautions.

To the fullest extent of the law, neither the Publisher nor the authors, contributors, or editors assume any liability for any injury and/or damage to persons or property as a matter of products liability, negligence or otherwise, or from any use or operation of any methods, products, instructions, or ideas contained in the material herein.

ISBN: 978-0-323-08498-7

Vice President and Publisher: Andrew Allen
Executive Content Strategist: Jennifer Janson
Senior Content Development Specialist: Kelly Brinkman
Publishing Services Manager: Hemamalini Rajendrababu
Project Manager: Prathibha Mehta

Printed in United States of America

Last digit is the print number: 9 8 7 6 5 4 3

Working together to grow
libraries in developing countries

www.elsevier.com | www.bookaid.org | www.sabre.org

ELSEVIER   BOOK AID
             International

D1449859

Workbook for

Pharmacology for Pharmacy Technicians

Second Edition

Prepared by:

Bobbi Steelman, CPhT, BSEd, MAEd, Rank 1
School Administration
Pharmacy Technology Program Director
Daymar College
Bowling Green, Kentucky

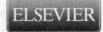

Preface

The goal of this workbook is to help students apply and master key concepts and skills presented in *Pharmacology for Pharmacy Technicians*, 2nd edition. The exercises in this workbook reinforce comprehension of material from the textbook.

The following exercises provide a sufficient review of concepts and allow students to apply the concepts from the text:

- Each chapter begins with a matching exercise of the **terms and definitions** in the text.
- **Fill-in-the-Blank** questions allow the student to review generic and brand name drugs.

- A variety of question formats test knowledge of concepts in the book, including **matching, multiple choice, and true/false**.
- **Critical thinking** exercises require students to use the knowledge they have learned in the chapter and apply it to specially designed exercises.
- **Research Activities** allow students to take the concepts they have learned and do additional research on various topics.

Best wishes as you begin your journey to become a pharmacy technician!

Table of Contents

Fundamentals of Pharmacology

TERMS AND DEFINITIONS

Match each term with the correct definition below. Some terms may not be used.

A. Biopharmaceutical

B. Bioavailability

C. Controlled substance

D. Dose

E. Dosage forms

F. Dosing schedule

G. Drug

H. Drug delivery system

I. Enteral

J. Homeopathic medicine

K. Legend drug

L. Materia medica

M. Over-the-counter drug

N. Parenteral

O. Pharmacognosy

P. Pharmacology

Q. Pharmacotherapy

R. Toxicology

   1. The study of the biological, biochemical features of drugs of plant and animal origins is called _____.

   2. _____ is defined as the study of drugs and their interactions with living systems, including chemical and physical properties, toxicology, and therapeutics.

3. A(n) _____ is defined as a substance that is used to diagnose, treat, cure, prevent, or mitigate disease in humans or other animals.

4. A(n) _____ drug is administered orally, whereas a(n) _____ drug is administered by injection or infusion.

5. A(n) _____ may be obtained without a prescription, whereas a(n) _____ may only be obtained by prescription.

6. _____ is a Latin term meaning medicinal materials.

7. Medicines are formulated into many different _____ (formulations) and _____ that are designed to release a specific amount of drug.

8. A drug may be classified as a(n) _____ to restrict its possession because of its potential for abuse.

9. The term used to describe the use of drugs for the treatment of disease is _____.

10. The _____ is the frequency that the drug is administered (e.g., "four times a day").

11. A drug that is produced by the process of bioengineering involving recombinant DNA technology is classified as a(n) _____.

12. _____ is the science dealing with the study of poisons.

13. The term used to describe the extent to which a drug reaches the site of action and is available to produce its effects is _____.

14. _____ are drugs that are administered in minute quantities and stimulate natural body healing systems.

MULTIPLE CHOICE

1. All of the following statements about pharmacy technicians who have a working knowledge of pharmacology are true *except* _____.
   A. pharmacy technicians' work performance will be more accurate and efficient.
   B. pharmacy technicians may be able to reduce dispensing errors.
   C. more time will be spent searching for drugs when pharmacy technicians have good brand/generic name recognition.
   D. the selection of appropriate warning labels (auxiliary labels) to place on prescription vials of dispensed medicines is made easier.
   E. pharmacy technicians understand the importance of alerting the pharmacy to drug interactions, therapeutic duplication, and excessive dose alerts screened by the computer.

2. People from around the globe have contributed to the knowledge of drugs, including people from _____.
   A. Africa
   B. Asia
   C. Europe
   D. North and South America
   E. all of the above

3. Select the **false** statement. _____
   A. Papyrus Ebers was found in Egypt and is thought to be a copy of an ancient manuscript that dates to 3000 BC.
   B. Papyrus Ebers describes more than 700 medical compounds and lists more than 811 prescriptions.
   C. Castor oil is described in Papyrus Ebers.
   D. Tinctura opii is described in Papyrus Ebers.
   E. Aspirin is described in Papyrus Ebers.

4. Select the **false** statement regarding synthetic and naturally derived drugs. _____
   A. A naturally derived drug may be a chemical modification of a synthetic drug.
   B. A synthetic drug may be manufactured entirely from chemical ingredients unrelated to a natural drug.
   C. Plants have been collected, cultivated, and harvested for their healing properties and used in the treatment of illness.
   D. Natural drugs may be derived from plants, animals, or minerals.

5. Select the **true** statement. _____
   A. The official name of a drug is the brand name.
   B. The proprietary name, or brand name, is assigned by the regulatory authority responsible for licensing the drug.
   C. Factors considered when selecting a suitable proprietary name are (1) whether an existing drug has a look-alike or sound-alike name and (2) whether the generic name can be easily associated with the name of an active ingredient in the new drug.
   D. The chemical name is the same as the generic name of the drug.

6. All of the statements about generic drugs are true *except* _____.
   A. a generic drug contains the same active ingredient as the original manufacturer's drug.
   B. a generic drug and its brand name equivalent have the same strength of the active ingredient and the same dosage form.
   C. generic drugs are more expensive than brand name drugs.
   D. a generic drug may contain different inactive ingredients than the brand name product.

7. Oral administration is safe, easy, and _____.
   A. generally less economical than parenteral administration.
   B. generally more economical than parenteral administration.
   C. can include tablets, suppositories, and syrups.
   D. none of the above are correct.

8. All of the following statements about the preparation and administration of parenterally administered drugs are true *except* _____.
   A. aseptic technique must be used when preparing drugs for parenteral administration.
   B. high doses of drugs administered intravenously (injected into a vein) must be injected rapidly to avoid destruction of red blood cells (hemolysis).
   C. drugs formulated for intramuscular administration (injected into a muscle) may produce a rapid onset or a slow onset of action.
   D. parenteral formulations may be administered intravenously, intramuscularly, or subcutaneously.

9. Select the drug formulation that has a slow onset of action and prolonged effects. _____
   A. Inhalation (e.g., metered-dose inhaler)
   B. Sublingual tablet (e.g., nitroglycerin)
   C. Intramuscular depot injection (e.g., prolixin decanoate)
   D. All of the above

10. Examples of drugs that are formulated for transdermal use include all of the following *except* _____.
    A. nitroglycerin
    B. estrogen
    C. testosterone
    D. antibiotics

MATCHING

Match the U.S. legislation with its intended effect.

1. The _____ requires that all drugs be safe and effective before they are made available to the public.

2. The _____ is the first significant legislation passed to protect the public from harmful and ineffective drugs.

3. The _____ encouraged the creation of generic drugs.

4. The _____ established the distinction between legend drugs and over-the-counter drugs.

A. Durham-Humphrey amendment

B. Kefauver-Harris amendment

C. Drug Price Competition and Patent Term Restoration Act (1984)

D. Pure Food and Drug Act (1906)

TRUE OR FALSE

1. _____ Egypt, Mesopotamia, India, and China have contributed to our body of knowledge of medicinals.

2. _____ A synthetic drug may be a chemical modification of a natural drug or manufactured entirely from chemical ingredients.

3. _____ The Drug Enforcement Agency regulates the new drug and investigational new drug process in the United States.

4. _____ The Health Products and Food Branch of Health Canada regulates the use of therapeutic drugs in Canada.

5. _____ The new drug application process includes preclinical research; clinical studies; phase 1, 2, and 3 trials; and postmarket safety studies.

6. _____ The name of a new drug is made according to standards set by the Food and Drug Administration.

7. _____ In the United States, patent holders for new drugs are given up to 20 years' exclusive rights to manufacture and distribute the drugs.

8. _____ All drugs are formulated for delivery by mouth, injection, inhalation, or topical application to skin or a mucous membrane.

9. _____ The major routes of drug administration are enteral (oral), parenteral (intravenous, intramuscular, or subcutaneous), inhalation, and topical.

10. _____ Parenteral drugs with rapid onset of action are typically prepared in water-soluble solutions, and slow-onset, prolonged-duration-of-action formulations are suspended in oil or other nonaqueous vehicles (solvents).

CRITICAL THINKING

1. Why is it crucial for pharmacy technicians to practice aseptic technique when preparing drugs for parenteral administration?

_____

_____

_____

_____

_____

RESEARCH ACTIVITY

1. Conduct an Internet search of risk management plans to answer the following question: In Europe, manufacturers of new drugs must submit a risk management plan (EU-RMP) with their application for licensing. How might this practice help protect public health?

_____

_____

_____

_____

2 Principles of Pharmacology

TERMS AND DEFINITIONS

Match each term with the correct definition below. Some terms may not be used.

A. Absorption

B. Biotransformation

C. Bioavailability

D. Distribution

E. Duration of action

F. Diffusion

G. Enzymes

H. First-pass effect

I. Half-life

J. Hydrophobic

K. Ionization

L. Hydrophilic

M. Lipid

N. Lipophilic

O. Metabolism

P. Metabolite

Q. Peak effect

R. Pharmacokinetics

S. Prodru

1. Osmosis is an example of the process of _____, which is the passive movement of molecules across cell membranes from an area of high drug concentration to an area of lower drug concentration.

2. The cytochrome P-450 system consists of _____ capable of increasing the metabolism of drugs in the liver.

3. A product of metabolism, a _____ may be an inactivated drug or active drug with equal or greater activity than the parent drug.

4. The length of time it takes for the plasma concentration of an administered drug to be reduced by half is known as the _____ .

5. _____ is the chemical process involving the release of a proton (H^+). Ionized drug molecules may have a positive or negative charge.

6. Lipid-loving substances (_____) are _____ (water hating).

7. The extent to which a drug reaches the site of action and is available to produce its effects is termed _____.

8. A _____ is a drug that is administered in an inactive form and metabolized in the body to an active form.

9. _____ drugs are water loving.

10. During the pharmacokinetic phase of _____, the drug undergoes _____, a process whereby the drug is converted to a more active, equally active, or inactive metabolite.

11. The first pharmacokinetic phase is _____, the process involving the movement of drug molecules from the site of administration into the circulatory system.

12. The _____ is the process whereby the liver metabolizes nearly all of a drug before it passes into the general circulation.

13. The maximum effect produced by a drug is known as the _____ and is achieved once the drug has reached its maximum concentration in the body.

14. _____ is the science dealing with the dynamic process a drug undergoes to produce its therapeutic effect.

15. A(n) _____ is a fatlike substance.

16. The process of movement of a drug from the circulatory system across barrier membranes to the site of drug action is called _____.

17. _____ is the time between the onset and discontinuation of drug action.

MULTIPLE CHOICE

1. Which of the following may be substituted for the brand name drug when authorized (i.e., follows product substitution laws)? _____
   A. Pharmaceutical alternative drug
   B. Pharmaceutical equivalent drug
   C. Bioequivalent drug
   D. Therapeutic alternative drug

2. Which of the following is *not* a pharmacokinetic phase? _____
   A. Disintegration
   B. Absorption
   C. Distribution
   D. Metabolism
   E. Elimination

3. The time it takes a drug to reach the concentration necessary to produce a therapeutic effect is the

_____.
   A. site of action
   B. duration of action
   C. onset of action
   D. mechanism of action

4. The rate of absorption depends on the

_____.
   A. lipid solubility
   B. extent of ionization
   C. surface area
   D. all of the above
   E. none of the above

5. Name the process that describes the movement of a drug from the circulatory system to its site

of action. _____
   A. Absorption
   B. Distribution
   C. Metabolism
   D. Excretion

6. The pharmacist tells Mr. Hsu that various patient factors may influence renal elimination, such as

the _____.
   A. pH of the urine
   B. patient's weight
   C. route of administration
   D. patient's gender

7. Oral administration is safe, easy, and

_____.
   A. administered by an intravenous line
   B. generally more economical than parenteral administration
   C. more effective
   D. none of the above

8. How are parenteral medications administered?

_____
   A. Intravenously and intrathecally
   B. Intravenously only
   C. Orally and intravenously
   D. None of the above

9. The main organ for metabolism is the

_____.
   A. kidney
   B. liver
   C. heart
   D. stomach

10. Metabolism of a drug can result in

_____.
   A. converting a prodrug to its active form
   B. converting an active drug to an inactive metabolite
   C. converting an active drug to a more active metabolite
   D. all of the above
   E. none of the above

11. Premature infants are especially sensitive to drugs because of all of the following *except*

_____.
   A. their kidneys are not well developed
   B. their drug-metabolizing capacity is limited
   C. their capacity for protein binding of drugs is excessive
   D. their lungs are not well developed

MATCHING

1. A _____ contains the same active ingredient as the brand name drug; however, the strength and dosage form may be different.

2. A _____ shows no statistical differences in the rate and extent of absorption when it is administered in the same strength, dosage form, and route of administration as the brand name product.

3. A _____ contains an identical amount of active ingredient as the brand name drug but may have different inactive ingredients or be manufactured in a different dosage form.

4. A _____ contains different active ingredient(s) than the brand name drug yet produces the same desired therapeutic outcome.

A. bioequivalent drug

B. pharmaceutical alternative

C. pharmaceutical equivalent

D. therapeutic alternative

MATCHING

1. _____ Water loving   A. Hydrophobic

2. _____ Water hating   B. Lipophobic

3. _____ Lipid loving   C. Hydrophilic

4. _____ Lipid hating   D. Lipophilic

TRUE OR FALSE

1. _____ Hydrophobic drugs dissolve readily in water.

2. _____ A synthetic drug may be a chemical modification of a natural drug or manufactured entirely from chemical ingredients.

3. _____ The first-pass effect describes why some drugs, if taken orally, would be inactivated before exerting an effect.

4. _____ Protein-bound drugs pass easily through capillary walls.

5. _____ Factors influencing metabolism are kidney function, disease, patient age, drug interactions, genetics, nutrition, and patient gender.

6. _____ The pharmaceutical phase of drug disposition involves drug disintegration and absorption.

7. _____ Drugs are absorbed across cell membranes via active and passive transport mechanisms.

CRITICAL THINKING

1. Compare and contrast pharmaceutical alternatives, pharmaceutical equivalents, bioequivalent drugs, and therapeutic alternatives. Relate your discussion to generic substitution.

_____

_____

_____

_____

_____

RESEARCH ACTIVITY

1. We typically think of drug interactions as bad. Conduct an Internet search of drug interactions to find examples of drugs that are administered concurrently for the beneficial effects of their interaction.

_____

_____

_____

_____

_____

2. How can pharmacy technicians help reduce harmful drug interactions?

_____

_____

_____

_____

_____

3 Pharmacodynamics

TERMS AND DEFINITIONS

Match each term with the correct definition below. Some terms may not be used.

A. Affinity

B. Drug-receptor theory

C. Efficacy

D. Hepatoxicity

E. Idiosyncratic reaction

F. Mechanism of action

G. Nephrotoxicity

H. Pharmacodynamics

I. Pharmacotherapeutics

J. Potency

K. Receptor site

L. Therapeutic index

M. Agonist

N. Partial agonist

O. Inverse agonist

P. Antagonist

Q. Noncompetitive antagonist

1. _____ is the study of drugs and their actions on a living organism.

2. _____ is a serious adverse effect that may occur in the kidney.

3. A drug must interact or bind with targeted cells, according to _____, for drug action to be produced.

4. _____ is a serious adverse reaction that occurs in the liver.

5. An unexpected drug reaction is known as a(n) _____.

6. The use of drugs in the treatment of disease, _____, is the study of factors that influence the patient response to drugs.

7. The _____ is a ratio of the effective dose to the lethal dose.

8. _____ is the measure of a drug's effectiveness.

9. _____ is defined as the effective dose concentration.

10. _____ is defined as the attraction that the _____ has for the drug.

11. The manner in which a drug produces its effect is the _____.

12. The drug that can turn "off" an activated receptor and turn "on" a receptor not currently active is known as a(n) _____.

13. _____ is a drug that binds to its receptor site and stimulates a cellular response.

14. A drug that binds to an alternative receptor site that prevents binding of an agonist is a(n) _____.

15. Binding drugs that do not produce action are known as _____.

16. A(n) _____ behaves as an agonist under some conditions and acts as an antagonist under other conditions.

MULTIPLE CHOICE

1. Select the statement about drug-receptor binding that is **false**. _____
   A. The more similar a drug is to the shape of a receptor site, the greater is the affinity the receptor site has for the drug.
   B. Drug-receptor binding may enhance or inhibit normal biological processes.
   C. An agonist is a drug that binds to its receptor site and stimulates a cellular response.
   D. Antagonist binding turns off a receptor that was activated.
   E. Drug-receptor binding is like a "lock and key."

2. Individual variation in pharmacokinetic and pharmacological responses may be caused by all of the following *except* the patient's _____.
   A. weight and gender
   B. emotional state
   C. age
   D. disease state
   E. hair color

3. Patient David Grant has developed a seizure disorder after a head injury. His physician prescribes phenytoin 100 mg three times a day. When explaining the use of phenytoin in treating a seizure disorder to Mr. Grant, the pharmacist is explaining what aspect of drug therapy? _____
   A. Pharmacotherapeutics
   B. Pharmacodynamics
   C. Pharmacokinetics
   D. Pharmacology

4. Which drug is most potent? _____

   A. Drug A
   B. Drug B
   C. Drug C
   D. Drug D

5. The basic requirement of a receptor is

_____.
   A. recognition of molecules to bind and produce an effect in the cell
   B. that it fit only one drug
   C. that it is the place to deposit your genes
   D. none of the above

6. An elderly patient is likely to experience adverse drug reactions more frequently than an adolescent patient. Which factor primarily accounts for this?

_____
   A. Drug clearance is more rapid in adolescents.
   B. Elderly patients are more likely to be taking multiple drugs than adolescent patients, and, therefore, drug elimination is slower in elderly patients.
   C. Adolescent patients have increased blood flow to the gastrointestinal tract.
   D. Higher doses are given to geriatric patients.

7. Which statement about drug dependence is **false**?

_____
   A. Drug dependence is an adverse reaction that is associated with antibiotics.
   B. When dependence develops, a patient must take increasing doses of a drug to get the desired effect.
   C. When dependence has developed, a patient must continue to take a drug to prevent withdrawal symptoms.
   D. All drugs can produce dependence.

8. The drug butorphanol (Stadol) is an example of which of the following? _____
   A. Antagonist
   B. Inverse agonist
   C. Partial agonist
   D. Drug-receptor theory

9. Adherence to drug therapy can be improved when

_____.
   A. affordable medicines are prescribed
   B. drug dosing schedules are convenient and easy to follow
   C. prescribed drugs have few side effects
   D. a patient believes the drug therapy is beneficial
   E. all of the above

10. A pharmacy should report suspected adverse drug reactions to the _____.
   A. Drug Enforcement Agency (DEA)
   B. Food and Drug Administration (FDA)
   C. Centers for Disease Control and Prevention (CDC)
   D. board of pharmacy

MATCHING

1. A _____ is able to produce a serious adverse reaction in the liver.

2. A _____ is able to produce a serious reaction in the kidney.

3. A _____ is able to produce harm to a developing fetus.

4. A _____ is able to stimulate the growth of cancers.

   A. teratogen

   B. carcinogen

   C. hepatotoxic drug

   D. nephrotoxic drug

MATCHING

1. _____ Lethal dose for 50% of the population

2. _____ Maximum possible effect that could be produced

3. _____ Effective dose for 50% of the population

4. _____ Effective dose concentration

5. _____ Decreased drug response over time because of repeated exposure

   A. Ceiling effect

   B. Potency

   C. LD_{50}

   D. Desensitization

   E. ED_{50}

TRUE OR FALSE

1. _____ Drugs that are administered in very low doses yet produce a maximum effect have high efficacy.

2. _____ A steep dose-response curve indicates that a large change in a drug dose is required to produce a big change in the drug response.

3. _____ Safe drugs have a wide margin between the lethal dose and the effective dose.

4. _____ Age, gender, disease, pregnancy, weight, and genetics are patient-related factors that influence the drug response.

5. _____ The placebo effect demonstrates that only biological factors are responsible for the patient response to drugs.

6. _____ Extended-release medications decrease patient adherence.

7. _____ Patients may develop tolerance to the side effects of a drug without developing tolerance to its therapeutic effects.

CRITICAL THINKING

1. Draw a dose-response curve. (Label the maximum therapeutic drug level and the ceiling effect.)

2. Write a short paragraph describing the relationship between the receptor site, agonists, and antagonists.

_____

_____

_____

_____

_____

1. What can pharmacy technicians do to reduce the patient's risk for adverse drug reactions, within the scope of practice for technicians?

_____

_____

_____

_____

_____

4 Drug Interactions and Medication Errors

TERMS AND DEFINITIONS

Match each term with the correct definition below. Some terms may not be used.

A. Additive effect

B. Antagonism

C. Drug contraindication

D. Drug-drug interaction

E. Drug-food interaction

F. Drug-disease contraindication

G. Medication error

H. Potentiation

I. Synergistic effects

J. Therapeutic duplication

1. An error made in the process of prescribing, preparing, dispensing, or administering drug therapy is called a

   _____.

2. An altered drug response that occurs when a drug is administered with certain foods is called

   _____.

3. _____ is a condition under which a drug is not indicated and should not be administered.

4. Interactions between two drugs may produce _____ that are greater than would be produced if either drug were administered alone.

5. _____ is the administration of two drugs that produce similar effects and side effects.

6. _____ is a reaction that occurs when two or more drugs are administered at the same time.

7. When administration of the drug may worsen the patient's medical condition, a(n) _____ exists.

8. An increased drug effect, or _____, is produced when a second similar drug is added to therapy and the effects produced are greater than the effects produced by either drug alone.

9. _____ is a process by which one drug or food, acting at a separate site or via a different mechanism of action, increases the effect of another drug, yet produces no effect when administered alone.

10. A drug-drug interaction or drug-food interaction that causes decreased effects is called _____.

MULTIPLE CHOICE

1. A drug interaction that can increase the risk for pregnancy may occur when _____ is(are) taken with oral contraceptives.
   A. birth control pills
   B. amoxicillin
   C. aspirin
   D. antihistamines
   E. ibuprofen

2. Which of the following fruits is implicated in food-drug interactions? _____
   A. Apple
   B. Pear
   C. Grapefruit
   D. Plum
   E. Grape

3. Which vitamin may be administered as an antidote for the drug warfarin? _____
   A. Vitamin A
   B. Vitamin B
   C. Vitamin C
   D. Vitamin D
   E. Vitamin K

4. Which way of writing the milligram (mg) strength of a drug can reduce medication errors? _____
   A. 1.0 mg
   B. 1 mg
   C. 1.00 mg
   D. 01 mg

5. Which is *not* a characteristic of an "aseptic attitude" when preparing parenteral medications?
   _____
   A. Handwashing
   B. Hood cleaning
   C. Dose calculating
   D. Proper technique
   E. Eating in the clean room

6. Pharmacy technicians may reduce medication errors by all of the following *except* _____.
   A. always checking the original prescription against the prescription label and the NDC number (DIN number in Canada) on the stock bottle
   B. asking patients to spell sound-alike drugs when they call to request refills
   C. guessing what the medication might be when the handwriting on the prescription is difficult to read
   D. always placing a zero in front of the decimal point when calculating doses that are less than 1 mL or 1 mg.
   E. writing legibly

7. Medication errors that may be made by pharmacy technicians include all of the following *except*
   _____.
   A. bagging errors
   B. labeling errors
   C. product selection errors
   D. prescribing errors
   E. transcribing errors

8. Which statement about drug interactions is **false**?
   _____
   A. Drug interactions may be caused by induction or inhibition of metabolic enzymes.
   B. Interactions cannot be avoided by maintaining an up-to-date history of the patients' chronic and acute medical conditions.
   C. Interactions that involve competition for a common transport system in the kidney can affect the elimination of some drugs.
   D. Pharmacists and pharmacy technicians should screen all prescriptions for potential drug interactions before dispensing a medication.

9. When warfarin and _____ are administered together, excessive bleeding occurs.
   A. acetaminophen
   B. codeine
   C. penicillin
   D. aspirin

10. Which abbreviation can be found on the Joint Commission "Do Not Use" list? _____
    A. QD
    B. BID
    C. TID
    D. QID

MATCHING

1. _____ One dram

2. _____ Poor handwriting

3. _____ Ounce

4. _____ Zyprexa and Celexa

5. _____ No known drug allergies

A. "Chicken scratch"

B. "Sound-alike, look-alike" drug names

C. (ʒi)

D. NKDA

E. (ʒ)

TRUE OR FALSE

1. _____ The pharmacy should collect information about a patient's use of over-the-counter drugs and enter it into the patient profile.

2. _____ NKDA is an abbreviation commonly used in pharmacies that means the patient does not have drug allergies.

3. _____ Pharmacy technicians unfamiliar with apothecary symbols may confuse the symbols for ounce and dram.

4. _____ The more drugs that are administered to a patient, the less likely it is that interactions will occur.

5. _____ Coadministration of drugs and foods can increase absorption, distribution, metabolism, or elimination.

6. _____ The process by which a drug, or a food, increases the effects of another drug, yet does not produce any effects when administered alone, is called antagonism.

7. _____ Intravenous solutions of acids and bases are incompatible, and when the solutions are combined, solid particles (precipitates) form.

8. _____ Studies indicate that between 7% and 22% of adverse drug reactions are caused by drug-drug interactions.

9. _____ Preventable medication errors are the cause of nearly 89,000 deaths in the United States annually; this number exceeds deaths due to motor vehicle accidents, breast cancer, and AIDS.

10. _____ Medication errors associated with prescribers are often a result of carelessness.

CRITICAL THINKING

1. It is recommended that pharmacy technicians develop a routine to avoid medication errors associated with distractions. Write a routine for yourself that you believe will help you avoid making medication errors in the pharmacy.

_____

_____

_____

_____

_____

2. Complete the missing information in the chart below using your knowledge of dangerous abbreviations.

Abbreviation	Interpretation	Alternate interpretation
QD		
		Morphine sulphate
	Intravenous	
AU, AS, AD		
	Half-strength	
		Discontinue

RESEARCH ACTIVITY

1. Conduct an Internet search on medication errors. What is the scope of the problem in the United States and Canada? What are the costs to patients, the health care system, and society?

_____

_____

_____

_____

_____

5 | Treatment of Anxiety

TERMS AND DEFINITIONS

Match each term with the correct definition below. Some terms may not be used.

A. Anxiety

B. Anxiolytic

C. Drug dependence

D. Generalized anxiety disorder

E. Obsessive-compulsive disorder

F. Panic disorder

G. Phobia

H. Posttraumatic stress disorder

I. Tolerance

1. An irrational fear of things or situations, a(n) _____ produces symptoms of intense anxiety.

2. _____ is a condition associated with an inability to control or stop repeated unwanted thoughts or behaviors.

3. A stress disorder that develops in persons who have participated in, witnessed, or been a victim of a terrifying

   event is a called _____.

4. When a person must take increasing doses of a drug in order to achieve the same effects as were achieved at

   previously lower doses, he or she has developed _____.

5. _____ is a condition that is associated with excessive worrying and tension that is experienced daily for more than 6 months.

6. Repeated episodes of a sudden onset of feelings of terror are associated with _____.

7. A(n) _____ is a drug that is used to treat _____, a condition associated with tension, apprehension, fear, or panic.

8. When a person taking a drug must continue to take the drug in order to avoid the onset of physical and/or

   psychological withdrawal symptoms, he or she has developed _____.

9. _____ is a drug used to treat anxiety.

MULTIPLE CHOICE

1. Anxiety disorders are *not* linked to

    _____ factors.
    A. environmental
    B. societal
    C. biological
    D. developmental
    E. socioeconomic

2. All of the following are major types of anxiety

    disorders *except* _____.
    A. generalized anxiety disorder
    B. panic disorder
    C. depression
    D. obsessive-compulsive disorder
    E. posttraumatic stress disorder

3. Which of the following is *not* an accepted medical

    treatment for anxiety? _____
    A. Administration of anxiolytics
    B. Psychotherapy
    C. Cognitive-behavioral therapy
    D. Self-administration of alcohol

4. Select the **false** statement. _____
    A. Benzodiazepines may produce tolerance and
       dependence.
    B. Benzodiazepines may be long acting, intermediate
       acting, or short acting.
    C. Benzodiazepines may induce amnesia.
    D. Benzodiazepines close chloride (Cl)$^-$ ion
       channels.
    E. Benzodiazepines bind to receptor sites on the
       GABA$_A$ complex.

5. Which drug is *not* a benzodiazepine?

    _____
    A. Xanax
    B. Valium
    C. BuSpar
    D. clorazepate
    E. clonazepam

6. To which class schedule does Valium belong?

    _____
    A. 1
    B. 2
    C. 3
    D. 4
    E. 5

7. A warning label that should be affixed to prescription

    vials for buspirone is _____.
    A. MAY CAUSE DROWSINESS
    B. AVOID PROLONGED EXPOSURE TO
       SUNLIGHT
    C. SWALLOW WHOLE; DO NOT CRUSH OR
       CHEW
    D. AVOID ANTACIDS, DAIRY PRODUCTS, AND
       FE^{++} PRODUCTS
    E. TAKE WITH LOTS OF WATER

8. An additional warning label that should be affixed
   to prescription vials for benzodiazepines is

    _____.
    A. AVOID PROLONGED EXPOSURE TO SUN-
       LIGHT
    B. TAKE WITH LOTS OF WATER
    C. MAY BE HABIT FORMING
    D. AVOID ANTACIDS, DAIRY PRODUCTS,
       AND FE^{++}
       PRODUCTS

9. Which of the following anxiolytics is also an

    antihistamine? _____
    A. lorazepam
    B. diazepam
    C. clomipramine
    D. buspirone
    E. hydroxyzine HCl

10. Which pair of drugs used to treat anxiety does *not*
    produce tolerance or dependence?

    _____
    A. lorazepam and buspirone
    B. buspirone and hydroxyzine HCl
    C. hydroxyzine HCl and diazepam
    D. diazepam and alprazolam

FILL IN THE BLANK: DRUG NAMES

1. What is the *brand name* for alprazolam? _____

2. What is the *generic name* for Tranxene (United States)? _____

3. What is the *brand name* for clonazepam? _____

4. What is the *generic name* for Valium? _____

5. What is the *brand name* for lorazepam? _____

6. What is the *generic name* for Anafranil? _____

7. What is the *brand name* for buspirone? _____

8. What is the *generic name* for Cymbalta? _____

9. What is the *brand name* for paroxetine? _____

10. What is the *brand name* for hydroxyzine HCl? _____

11. What is the *generic name* for Prozac? _____

12. What is the *brand name* for sertraline? _____

MATCHING

Match each drug to its pharmacological classification.

1. _____ Clomipramine   A. Benzodiazepines

2. _____ BuSpar   B. Antidepressants

3. _____ Hydroxyzine HCl   C. Miscellaneous (antihistamine)

4. _____ Alprazolam   D. Azapirones

TRUE OR FALSE

1. _____ Anxiety disorders are the leading form of mental health illness.

2. _____ Xanax immediate-release tablets and extended-release tablets come in different strengths, so verification of the dosage form is never needed.

3. _____ A drug classified as a controlled substance IV does not pose a risk for tolerance and dependence.

4. _____ Symptoms of anxiety are associated with hyperactivity of the autonomic nervous system.

5. _____ Fear of public speaking is an example of obsessive-compulsive disorder.

6. _____ Benzodiazepines can produce an amnesia that causes the person receiving the drug to "forget," reducing anxiety associated with future medical procedures.

7. _____ Benzodiazepines are not capable of producing tolerance and dependence.

8. _____ Propranolol may be administered to reduce palpitations caused by stage fright.

The following hard copies are brought to your pharmacy for filling. Identify the prescription error(s). (You already have the patient's full address on file.)

```
Micheal Vessalago, MD      Date _____
         1221 Madison #310
         Anytown, USA

Pt. Name _____ Lillie Neville _____
Address _____

℞   buspirone #60
      i BID


Refills __6__
      Vessalago
_____      _____
Substitution permitted      Dispense as written
```

1. Spot the error in the following prescription:
   A. RF limit exceeded
   B. Incorrect dosage form
   C. Incorrect directions
   D. No strength written
   E. Quantity missing

```
Kathy Principi, MD      Date _____
         1145 Broadway
         Anytown, USA

Pt. Name _____ Ellen Wilbur-Jones _____
Address _____

℞   lorazepam 1mg
      1 tablet BID


Refills __1__
      Principi
_____      _____
Substitution permitted      Dispense as written
```

2. Spot the error in the following prescription:
   A. Quantity missing
   B. Strength incorrect
   C. Strength missing
   D. Directions incorrect
   E. Dosage form incorrect

```
Kathy Principi, MD      Date _____
         1145 Broadway
         Anytown, USA

Pt. Name _____ Preston Scott _____
Address _____

℞   clonazepam 25mg   #30
      1 BID for panic


Refills _____
      Principi
_____      _____
Substitution permitted      Dispense as written
```

3. Spot the error in the following prescription:
   A. Quantity missing
   B. Strength missing
   C. Strength incorrect
   D. Directions incorrect
   E. Dosage form incorrect

Chapter 5 **Treatment of Anxiety**

4. List six pairs of anxiolytic drugs that have look-alike or sound-alike issues.

DRUG NAME	LOOK-ALIKE OR SOUND-ALIKE DRUG

RESEARCH ACTIVITY

1. Access the National Library of Medicine website (nlm.nih.gov/medlineplus/anxiety) to identify and list nonpharmacological methods for reducing anxiety.

_____

_____

_____

_____

_____

6 Treatment of Depression

TERMS AND DEFINITIONS

Match each term with the correct definition below. Some terms may not be used.

A. Adjunct

B. Bipolar disorder

C. Enuresis

D. Major depression

E. Mood disorder

F. Monoamine oxidase

G. Serotonin syndrome

1. An affective disorder, or _____, involves a change in emotional behavior.

2. Bedwetting, or _____, is characterized by uncontrollable urination during sleep.

3. _____ is a potentially life-threatening adverse drug reaction caused by excessive serotonin.

4. A mental health illness associated with sudden swings in mood between depression and periods of insomnia, racing thoughts, and distractibility is _____.

5. _____ is a mental health illness associated with persistent feelings of sadness, emptiness, or hopelessness that persists for several weeks.

6. A drug is classified as _____ therapy when it is used to complement the effects of another drug.

7. _____ is an enzyme that is responsible for degradation of monoamine neurotransmitters and dietary amines.

MULTIPLE CHOICE

1. Clinical depression is caused by a

   _____.
   A. decrease in brain acetylcholine
   B. decrease in brain histamine
   C. decrease in brain serotonin, norepinephrine, and dopamine
   D. deficiency of certain neurotransmitters

2. Which drug classification is *not* used in the treatment of depression? _____
   A. Tricyclic antidepressants
   B. Benzodiazepines
   C. Monoamine oxidase inhibitors
   D. Selective serotonin reuptake inhibitors

3. Bipolar disorder is also known as _____.
   A. mania
   B. depression
   C. mood disorder
   D. none of the above

4. A blockade of histaminic receptors can lead to

   _____.
   A. hypertension and weight loss
   B. weight loss and insomnia
   C. hair loss and skin rash
   D. sedation, weight gain, and hypotension

5. Symptoms of bipolar disorder are _____.
   A. racing thoughts
   B. distractibility
   C. increased goal-directed behavior
   D. insomnia
   E. all of the above

6. The enzyme monoamine oxidase is found in all of

   the following sites *except* the _____.
   A. kidney
   B. liver
   C. intestines
   D. terminal neurons

7. Which adverse effects are *not* associated with

   serotonin syndrome? _____.
   A. Confusion and agitation
   B. Lethargy and drowsiness
   C. Diarrhea
   D. Tremors and seizures
   E. Increased blood pressure

8. The mechanism(s) of action of drugs used to treat

   clinical depression are _____.
   A. inhibition of reuptake monoamine
      neurotransmitters
   B. blocking of the degradation of monoamine
      neurotransmitters
   C. increasing the reuptake of monamine
      neurotransmitters
   D. inhibition of the reuptake of histamine
   E. A and C

9. Select the **false** statement about tricyclic

   antidepressants (TCAs). _____.
   A. TCAs are the oldest class of antidepressants.
   B. TCAs are cardiotoxic in some patients.
   C. TCAs specifically inhibit 5-hydroxytryptamine
      (5-HT).
   D. TCAs may cause dry mouth and increased
      cravings for sweets.
   E. TCAs should not be discontinued abruptly.

10. Select the drug that is *not* used in the treatment of

    bipolar disorder. _____.
    A. lithium
    B. paroxetine
    C. carbamazepine
    D. divalproex sodium
    E. lamotrigine

FILL IN THE BLANK: DRUG NAMES

1. What is the *generic name* for Tofranil? _____

2. What is the *brand name* for desipramine? _____

3. What is a *brand name* for doxepin? _____

4. What is a *brand name* for trimipramine? _____

5. What is a *brand name* for nortriptyline? _____

6. What is the *generic name* for Lexapro (United States)? _____

7. What is the *brand name* for citalopram? _____

8. What is the *generic name* for Prozac? _____

9. What is the *generic name* for Luvox? _____

10. What is the **brand name** for paroxetine? _____

11. What is the **generic name** for Zoloft? _____

12. What is the **brand name** for phenelzine? _____

13. What is the **generic name** for Parnate? _____

14. What is the **brand name** for bupropion? _____

15. What is the **brand name** for mirtazapine? _____

16. What is the **generic name** for Desyrel? _____

17. What is the **brand name** for venlafaxine? _____

18. What is a **brand name** for lithium carbonate? _____

19. What is the **brand name** for carbamazepine? _____

20. What is the **generic name** for Lamictal? _____

MATCHING

Patient education is an essential component of therapeutics. Select the **best** warning label to apply to the prescription vial given to patients taking the drugs listed.

1. _____ Nardil 10 mg

2. _____ Desyrel 50 mg

3. _____ Wellbutrin SR

4. _____ carbamazepine 100 mg

5. _____ amitriptyline 10 mg

A. MAY DISCOLOR URINE

B. SWALLOW WHOLE; DO NOT CRUSH OR CHEW

C. AVOID PREGNANCY

D. AVOID TYRAMINE-CONTAINING FOODS

E. TAKE WITH FOOD

MATCHING

Match each drug to its pharmacological classification.

1. _____ Prozac 20 mg

2. _____ phenelzine 15 mg

3. _____ venlafaxine XR 75 mg

4. _____ imipramine 10 mg

A. tricyclic antidepressant (TCA)

B. selective serotonin reuptake inhibitor (SSRI)

C. monoamine oxidase inhibitor (MAOI)

D. serotonin-noradrenaline reuptake inhibitor (SNRI)

MATCHING

Match each drug to its pharmacological classification.

1. _____ bupropion 150 mg SR

A. tricyclic antidepressant (TCA)

2. _____ desipramine 50 mg

B. selective serotonin reuptake inhibitor (SSRI)

3. _____ tranylcypromine

C. serotonin-noradrenaline reuptake inhibitor (SNRI)

4. _____ doxepin

D. noradrenaline-dopamine inhibitor (NA/DRI)

5. _____ paroxetine 20 mg

E. monoamine oxidase inhibitor (MAOI)

TRUE OR FALSE

1. _____ Tricyclic antidepressants (TCAs) can increase cravings for sweets.

2. _____ Prescriptions for large quantities of TCAs may be written for depressed patients who are believed to be suicidal.

3. _____ Lithium has a narrow therapeutic index.

4. _____ A hypertensive crisis is a fatal adverse reaction associated with TCAs.

5. _____ Prescriptions for MAOIs should be dispensed with a list of tyramine-containing foods and a list of drugs to avoid.

6. _____ Contents of Effexor-XR capsules cannot be sprinkled onto food.

7. _____ The endings -tyline and -pramine are commonly used for tricyclic antidepressants.

8. _____ A common ending for SSRIs is -oxetine.

9. _____ According to the biogenic amine theory, clinical depression results from an increase in monoamine neurotransmitters in the brain.

CRITICAL THINKING

The following hard copies are brought to your pharmacy for filling. Identify the prescription error(s). (You already have the patient's full address on file.)

```
Micheal Vessalago, MD     Date _____
         1221 Madison #310
         Anytown, USA

Pt. Name _____ Fatou Njie _____
Address _____ 2306 Broadway E Sea, WA _____

R̥  imipramine 10 mg, i qd x 3d, ii qd x 3d,
     iii qd x 3d, iv qd thereafter




Refills __5__
 Vessalago              _____
Substitution permitted      Dispense as written
```

1. Spot the error in the following prescription:

    _____

    A. Quantity missing

    B. Strength missing

    C. Strength incorrect

    D. Directions missing

    E. Dosage form incorrect

```
Kathy Principi, MD          Date _____
            1145 Broadway
            Anytown, USA
Pt. Name _____ Will Jones _____
Address _____
℞    amitriptyline 50mg tab    #30
     1 tablet


Refills _____
_____ Principi _____        _____
Substitution permitted        Dispense as written
```

2. Spot the error in the following prescription:

   _____

   A. Quantity missing
   B. Directions incomplete
   C. Strength missing
   D. Strength incorrect
   E. Dosage form incorrect

```
Anh Dang Tu, MD          Date _____
            1145 Broadway
            Anytown, USA
Pt. Name _____ Phuong Nguyen _____
Address _____
℞    Wellbutrin 150mg SR tab    #60
     i tab QID


Refills _____
_____ A. Tu _____           _____
Substitution permitted        Dispense as written
```

3. Spot the error in the following prescription:

   _____

   A. Quantity missing
   B. Strength missing
   C. Strength incorrect
   D. Directions incorrect
   E. Dosage form incorrect

```
Kathy Principi, MD          Date _____
            1145 Broadway
            Anytown, USA
Pt. Name _____ Preston Scott _____
Address _____
℞    fluoxetine capsules
     1 g AM


Refills _ 2 _
_____ Principi _____        _____
Substitution permitted        Dispense as written
```

4. Spot the error in the following

   prescription: _____

   A. Quantity missing
   B. Strength missing
   C. DEA number missing
   D. Directions incorrect
   E. Dosage form incorrect

5. Write a short paragraph comparing and contrasting the mechanisms of action of TCAs, SSRIs, and MAOIs.

   _____

   _____

   _____

   _____

   _____

6. How many tablets are required to fill Crystal Boelle's prescription for amitriptyline?

Amitriptyline 25 mg i QD x 3 days, ii QD x 3 days; iii QD x 3 days, iv QD thereafter.

Dispense a 1-month supply, and please show your calculations.

_____

_____

_____

_____

_____

7. List six pairs of antidepressant drugs that have look-alike or sound-alike issues.

DRUG NAME	LOOK-ALIKE OR SOUND-ALIKE DRUG

RESEARCH ACTIVITY

1. Sheila Bogan calls to refill her antidepressant medication. She does not remember the name. Review her patient profile, and make a list of the drugs used to treat depression. Search the Internet to find pictures of the drugs, and then develop a list of questions you might ask to identify the drug she is requesting.

Last Name: Bogan   First Name: Sheila   Gender: F

Address: 1310 34th Ave. S #310   City: Anytown   DOB: 12-14-53

Allergies: NKA   Disc: Phone: 725-2743

Insurance: PCS   Plan: 05   Group: 54873456

ID: 536234177   Copay: $10.00/$20.00

Cardholder: Kargan   Melinda   Exp. date:

DATE	RX#	DRUG AND STRENGTH	SIG	QTY	MD	RF
10-2-07	72345	amitriptyline 50 mg	1 HS	60	Johnson, C	2
11-1-07	72345	amitriptyline 50 mg	1 HS	60	Johnson, C	1
12-2-07	81956	meperidine 100 mg	1 q6h prn	20	Hohl DDS	0
12-2-07	84358	Anaprox DS	1 BID	30	Hohl DDS	1
1-2-08	85345	trazodone 50 mg	1 HS	30	Johnson, C	0
2-4-08	89278	Hycotuss	5-10 mL q6h	240	Johnson, C	3
2-4-08	96346	Paxil CR 25 mg	1 qd	30	Ng, A	2
3-12-08	102344	Darvocet N 100	1 q6h	25	Ng, A	1
3-12-08	102345	bupropion 150 mg SR	1 BID	60	Ng, A	1
4-4-08	102345	bupropion 150 mg SR	1 q12h	60	Johnson, C	2
5-4-08	103366	Effexor 75 mg XR	1 q12h	60	Johnson, C	1

Make a list of the antidepressant drugs listed in the profile.

Make a list of questions you might ask to identify the current drug she is requesting.

ANTIDEPRESSANT DRUG	DRUG IDENTIFICATION QUESTIONS
	1.
	2.
	3.

7 Treatment of Schizophrenia and Psychoses

TERMS AND DEFINITIONS

Match each term with the correct definition below. Some terms may not be used.

A. Catatonia

B. Delusion

C. Extrapyramidal symptoms

D. Hallucinations

E. Negative symptoms

F. Neuroleptic

G. Neuroleptic malignant syndrome

H. Positive symptoms

I. Postural hypotension

J. Pseudoparkinsonism

K. Psychosis

L. Schizophrenia

M. Tardive dyskinesia

1. A(n) _____ is a drug used to treat schizophrenia or other psychosis.

2. Potentially fatal, _____ produces symptoms such as stupor, muscle rigidity, and high temperature.

3. Persons with schizophrenia may exhibit _____ such as hallucinations, delusions, or other unusual thoughts.

4. A(n) _____ is a mental state characterized by disorganized behavior and thought, delusions, hallucinations, and a loss of touch with reality.

5. _____ is a symptom of schizophrenia that is associated with unresponsiveness and immobility.

6. The administration of neuroleptics may cause _____, excessive muscle movement, and difficulty in walking.

7. The term for a sudden drop in blood pressure upon a change in posture is _____.

8. The administration of neuroleptics may produce _____, an adverse reaction that mimics Parkinson's disease.

9. Persons with schizophrenia may have _____, irrational thoughts, or false beliefs that do not change even when evidence is provided that beliefs are not valid.

10. The administration of neuroleptics may produce _____, an adverse reaction that causes involuntary thrusting of the tongue and changes in posture.

11. Persons with schizophrenia may exhibit _____, which presents as a decreased ability to think, plan, or express emotion.

12. _____ is a type of psychosis characterized by delusions of thought, visual and/or auditory hallucinations, and speech disturbances.

13. Visions or voices that exist only in the mind and cannot be seen or heard by others are called _____.

MULTIPLE CHOICE

1. A neurotransmitter that has *not* been identified as playing a role in symptoms of schizophrenia is

   _____.
   A. dopamine
   B. serotonin
   C. GABA
   D. norepinephrine
   E. glutamate

2. Treatment for shizophrenia that involves dopamine

   blockade can produce_____.
   A. delusions
   B. neurolepsy
   C. psychosis
   D. pseudoparkinsonism

3. Paul Bunyan was institutionalized for schizophrenia. He was administered fluphenazine HCl, 2.5 mg IM every 6 hours, initially but has been switched to fluphenazine decanoate in preparation for discharge.

   Fluphenazine decanoate _____.
   A. is a slow-release preparation that is administered every 3 weeks
   B. should be dispensed with an oral syringe
   C. must be diluted in water or juice before administration
   D. is administered sublingually

4. Karen Linder is taking perphenazine, 8 mg twice a day. Which of the following warnings should she be

   given? _____
   A. MAY CAUSE DROWSINESS; ALCOHOL MAY INTENSIFY THIS EFFECT
   B. TAKE ON AN EMPTY STOMACH
   C. MAY BE HABIT FORMING
   D. TAKE WITH FOOD

5. Patients receiving chlorpromazine oral concentrate, 100 mg/mL, should be given the following

   advice: _____
   A. MAY CAUSE DROWSINESS OR DIZZINESS
   B. AVOID ALCOHOL
   C. DILUTE WITH LIQUID BEFORE INGESTION
   D. AVOID PROLONGED EXPOSURE TO SUN-LIGHT
   E. all of the above

6. Serious adverse reactions associated with the administration of neuroleptics include all of the following

   except _____.
   A. tardive dyskinesia
   B. delusions
   C. extrapyramidal symptoms
   D. neuroleptic malignant syndrome

7. Which statement about functional classifications

   for neuroleptics is **true**? _____
   A. High-potency neuroleptics have a weak affinity for dopamine receptors.
   B. "Atypical" neuroleptics have a strong affinity for dopamine receptors.
   C. Low-potency neuroleptics have a strong affinity for dopamine receptors.
   D. Low-potency and "atypical" neuroleptics produce fewer side effects.

8. A prototype for atypical neuroleptics is

   _____.
   A. clozapine
   B. chlorpromazine
   C. perphenazine
   D. haloperidol
   E. thiothixene

9. Up to _____ of the people who are prescribed neuroleptics will experience adverse reactions.
   A. 20%
   B. 40%
   C. 60%
   D. 80%
   E. 100%

10. Clozapine use is restricted because this drug can produce a fatal drop in the _____.
    A. white blood cell level
    B. red blood cell level
    C. blood pressure
    D. pulse

FILL IN THE BLANK: DRUG NAMES

1. What is the *generic name* for Invega (United States)? _____

2. What is the *generic name* for Prolixin Decanoate (United States) and Modecate (Canada)?

   _____

3. What is a *brand name* for olanzapine? _____

4. What is the *generic name* for Navane? _____

5. What is a *generic name* for Abilify? _____

6. What is the *brand name* for risperidone? _____

7. What is the *brand name* for fluphenazine? _____

8. What is a *brand name* for quetiapine? _____

9. What is the *generic name* for Clozaril (United States) and Clopsine (Canada)? _____

10. What is the *generic name* for Geodon (United States)? _____

11. What is the *generic name* for Loxitane (United States)? _____

MATCHING

Match each drug to its pharmacological classification.

1. _____ Navane

2. _____ clozapine

3. _____ Zyprexa

4. _____ trifluoperazine

5. _____ Risperdal

A. phenothiazines

B. benzoxazoles

C. thioxanthenes

D. dibenzodiazepines

E. thienobenzodiazepines

TRUE OR FALSE

1. _____ Haloperidol and risperidone oral concentrates should not be mixed with coffee or tea.

2. _____ Patients, prescribers, and pharmacists must be enrolled in a registry to dispense clozapine.

3. _____ The dropper that comes packaged with oral concentrate may be interchanged with other droppers and dispensed with the medicine.

4. _____ The greater the affinity a neuroleptic drug has for dopamine (D_2) receptors, the less effective is the drug.

CRITICAL THINKING

The following hard copies are brought to your pharmacy for filling. Identify the prescription error(s). (You already have the patient's full address on file.)

```
┌─────────────────────────────────────────────┐
│         Micheal Vessalago, MD    Date _____  │
│             1221 Madison #310                 │
│               Anytown, USA                    │
│                                               │
│ Pt. Name _____ G.W. Bushe _____ │
│ Address _____  │
│ Rx    Zyprexa    #30                          │
│         10mg daily                            │
│                                               │
│                                               │
│ Refills __3__                                 │
│      Vessalago                  _____  │
│ Substitution permitted     Dispense as written│
└─────────────────────────────────────────────┘
```

1. Spot the error in the following prescription:

   _____

   A. Quantity missing
   B. Strength missing
   C. Strength incorrect
   D. Directions missing
   E. Dosage form incorrect

```
┌─────────────────────────────────────────────┐
│          Anh Dang Tu, MD      Date _____     │
│             1145 Broadway                     │
│              Anytown, USA                     │
│                                               │
│ Pt. Name _____ Lili Ng _____ │
│ Address _____  │
│ Rx   Prolixin decanoate 25mg/ml               │
│      0.5 ml IM BID                             │
│      10ml                                      │
│ Refills __1__                                 │
│      A. Tu                      _____  │
│ Substitution permitted     Dispense as written│
└─────────────────────────────────────────────┘
```

2. Spot the error in the following prescription:

   _____

   A. Quantity missing
   B. Strength missing
   C. Strength incorrect
   D. Directions incorrect
   E. Dosage form incorrect

```
        Kathy Principi, MD      Date _____
           1145 Broadway
           Anytown, USA
Pt. Name _____ Preston Scott _____
Address _____
R̶x   Risperdal 1mg
        i bid x 1d; ii bid 2d; iii bid



Refills _____
____ Principi _____      _____
Substitution permitted          Dispense as written
```

3. Spot the error in the following prescription:

   _____

   A. Quantity missing
   B. Strength missing
   C. DEA number missing
   D. Directions incorrect
   E. Dosage form incorrect

4. List three pairs of examples of neuoroleptic drugs that have sound-alike or look-alike issues.

DRUG NAME	LOOK-ALIKE OR SOUND-ALIKE DRUG

5. Susan Kraft has been prescribed haloperidol, 2.5 mg twice a day. The pharmacy stocks 0.5-mg tablets. How many tablets will she need to take per day? Please show your calculations.

   _____

   _____

   _____

   _____

   _____

6. Nick Harper has previously been taking chlorpromazine, 50 mg PO every 6 hours. He has recently been hospitalized, and his medication has been changed from an oral to an intramuscular preparation (50 mg IM every 6 hours). Chlorpromazine HCl for parenteral use is available as 25 mg/mL. How many milliliters will you need to draw up into each syringe and send to his nursing unit? Please show your calculations.

   _____

   _____

   _____

   _____

   _____

1. Sheila Bogan calls to refill her medication. She does not remember the name. Review her patient profile, and make a list of the neuroleptic medications. Search the Internet to find pictures of the drugs, and then develop a list of questions you might ask to identify the drug she is requesting.

Last Name: Bogan	First Name: Sheila	Gender: F
Address: 1310 34th Ave. S #310	City: Anytown	DOB: 12-14-53
Allergies: NKA	Disc:	Phone: 725-2743
Insurance: PCS	Plan: 05	Group: 54873456
ID: 536234177	Copay: $10.00/$20.00	
Cardholder: Kargan	Melinda	Exp. date:

DATE	RX#	DRUG AND STRENGTH	SIG	QTY	MD	RF
10-2-07	72345	fluphenazine 5 mg	1 q8h	90	Johnson, C	2
11-1-07	72345	fluphenazine 5 mg	1 q8h	90	Johnson, C	1
12-2-07	81956	meperidine 100 mg	1 q6h prn	20	Hohl DDS	0
12-2-07	84358	Anaprox DS	1 BID	30	Hohl DDS	1
1-2-08	85345	fluphenazine 25 mg/mL	12.5 mg q3wk	5 mL	Johnson, C	0
1-21-08	85345	fluphenazine 25 mg/mL	12.5 mg q3wk	5 mL	Johnson, C	0
2-4-08	89278	Hycotuss	5-10 mL q6h	240 mL	Johnson, C	3
2-4-08	96346	Risperdal 2 mg	1 BID	60	Ng, A	2
3-3-08	96346	Risperdal 2 mg	1 BID	60	Ng, A	1
4-2-08	102345	Risperdal 3 mg	1 BID	60	Ng, A	1
5-1-08	103366	Zyprexa Zydis 5 mg	2 daily	60	Johnson, C	1

Make a list of neuroleptic drugs contained in the profile. Make a list of questions you might ask to identify the current drug she is requesting.

NEUROLEPTIC DRUG	DRUG IDENTIFICATION QUESTIONS
	1.
	2.
	3.

8 Treatment of Parkinson's Disease and Huntington's Disease

TERMS AND DEFINITIONS

Match each term with the correct definition below. Some terms may not be used.

A. Acetylcholinesterase

B. Basal ganglia

C. Bradykinesia

D. Cognitive function

E. Huntington's disease

F. Nigrostriatal pathways

G. Neurodegenerative diseases

H. Substantia nigra

I. Pseudoparkinsonism

J. Parkinson's disease

1. _____ are disorders that result from the progressive destruction of neurons.

2. The ability to take in information via the senses, process the details, commit the information to memory, and recall it when necessary is a(n) _____.

3. The enzyme that degrades the neurotransmitter acetylcholine is called _____.

4. The part of the basal ganglia that contains clusters of dopamine-producing neurons is called the _____.

5. _____ are located in the substantia nigra and stimulate and inhibit movement.

6. The subcortical nuclei located in the forebrain and brainstem called _____ initiate, control, and modulate movement and posture.

7. _____ is a drug-induced condition that resembles Parkinson's disease.

8. The term used to describe slowness in initiating and carrying out voluntary movements is _____.

9. _____ and _____ are progressive disorders of the nervous system that impair muscle movement.

MULTIPLE CHOICE

1. What is Parkinson's disease? _____
   A. A progressive and degenerative disease in newborns
   B. A drug-induced condition
   C. A disease resulting from a vitamin deficiency
   D. A progressive disorder of the nervous system

2. Entacapone and tolcapone are COMT inhibitors and boost the bioavailability of levodopa by

   _____.
   A. 10%
   B. 50%
   C. 0.5%
   D. 75%

3. At least _____ million people in the United States have Parkinson's disease.
   A. 5
   B. 10
   C. 2
   D. 1.2

4. Cholinergic receptors are located at the neuromuscular junction, at parasympathetic synapses, and in the brain and spinal cord. What are two types of

   cholinergic receptors? _____
   A. Nicotinic and basal ganglia
   B. Nicotinic and muscarinic
   C. Basal ganglia and muscarinic
   D. Depolarization and nicotinic

5. All of the following can be used to treat Parkinson's

   disease except _____.
   A. Duodopa
   B. Levodopa
   C. bromocriptine
   D. Miralax

6. Which adverse effect is not associated with

   anticholinergic drugs? _____
   A. Dry mouth
   B. Diarrhea
   C. Blurred vision
   D. Constipation
   E. Urinary retention

7. Huntington's disease differs from Parkinson's

   disease because _____.
   A. Huntington's disease is a progressive and degenerative disease of neurons
   B. Huntington's disease affects muscle movement, cognitive functions, and emotions
   C. Huntington's disease is primarily treated with drugs that decrease excessive dopaminergic activity
   D. Huntington's disease symptoms are caused by an imbalance between neurotransmitters (e.g., acetylcholine, dopamine, and GABA)

8. Parkinson's disease is treated with

   _____.
   A. pharmaceuticals
   B. exercise
   C. nutritional support
   D. all of the above

9. Huntington's disease is primarily treated with drugs

   that decrease excessive _____ activity.
   A. cholinergic
   B. acetylcholinesterase
   C. dopaminergic
   D. norepinephrine

10. Which of the following drugs is indicated for the treatment of Huntington's disease, Tourette's

    syndrome, and schizophrenia? _____
    A. Requip
    B. Xenazine
    C. Nitroman
    D. haloperidol

FILL IN THE BLANK: DRUG NAMES

1. What is the **brand name** for amantadine? _____

2. What is a **brand name** for bromocriptine? _____

3. What is the **generic name** for Stalevo (United States)? _____

4. What is a **brand name** for levodopa and carbidopa? _____

5. What is a **generic name** for Mirapex? _____

6. What is the **generic name** for Requip? _____

7. What is the **brand name** for selegiline? _____

8. What is a **brand name** for benztropine? _____

9. What is the **generic name** for Tasmar (United States)? _____

10. What is a **brand name** for tetrabenazine? _____

MATCHING

Match each drug to its pharmacological classification or brand or generic name.

1. _____ haloperidol   A. Xenazine

2. _____ tetrabenazine   B. benztropine

3. _____ Cogentin   C. tolcapone

4. _____ dopamine precursor   D. Haldol

5. _____ COMT inhibitor   E. levodopa

MATCHING

Patient education is an essential component of therapeutics. Select the **best** warning label to apply to the prescription vial given to patients taking the drugs listed.

1. _____ Sinemet 25 mg/100 mg   A. MAY CAUSE DIZZINESS; MAY IMPAIR ABILITY TO DRIVE

2. _____ bromocriptine   B. AVOID VITAMINS AND IRON SUPPLEMENTS WITHIN 2 HOURS OF DOSE

3. _____ Cogentin 0.5 mg

4. _____ Tasmar 100 mg   C. TAKE WITH FOOD

                                    D. MAY DISCOLOR URINE

TRUE OR FALSE

1. _____ Bradykinesia will speed up voluntary movements.

2. _____ The substantia nigra is a part of the basal ganglia containing clusters of dopamine-producing neurons.

3. _____ Cognitive functions are not involved in the ability to take information in via the senses, process the details, commit the information to memory, or recall the information when necessary.

4. _____ About 2 million people in the United States have Parkinson's disease.

5. _____ The prevalence of Parkinson's disease is greater in men than in women.

The following hard copies are brought to your pharmacy for filling. Identify the prescription error(s). (You already have the patient's full address on file.)

Micheal Vessalago, MD   Date _____
1221 Madison #310
Anytown, USA

Pt. Name _____ Marge Simpson _____

Address _____

℞   Parlodel 2.5mg
      1 tab q 12 h

Refills ___6___

_____Vessalago_____   _____
Substitution permitted   Dispense as written

---

1. Spot the error in the following prescription:

   _____

   A. Quantity missing
   B. Strength missing
   C. Strength incorrect
   D. Directions missing
   E. Dosage form incorrect

Kathy Principi, MD   Date _____
1145 Broadway
Anytown, USA

Pt. Name _____ Homer Wollensky _____

Address _____

℞   Levodopa/carbidopa   #90
      1 tab TID

Refills _PRN_

_____Principi_____   _____
Substitution permitted   Dispense as written

---

2. Spot the error in the following prescription:

   _____

   A. Quantity missing
   B. Directions incomplete
   C. Strength missing
   D. Strength incorrect
   E. Dosage form incorrect

Marc Cordova, MD   Date _____
1145 Broadway
Anytown, USA

Pt. Name _____ Bill Carey _____

Address _____

℞   Benztropine 0.5mg tab q 12 hours

Refills _____

_____Cordova_____   _____
Substitution permitted   Dispense as written

---

3. Spot the error in the following prescription:

   _____

   A. Quantity missing
   B. Directions incomplete
   C. Strength missing
   D. Strength incorrect
   E. Dosage form incorrect

---

4. Draw a picture to show the changes that occur in neurotransmitter levels in Parkinson's disease. BE SURE TO LABEL THE DIAGRAMS.

WITHOUT PARKINSON'S DISEASE	WITH PARKINSON'S DISEASE

5. List two pairs of drug names that have look-alike or sound-alike issues with drugs used to treat Parkinson's disease or Huntington's disease.

DRUG NAME	LOOK-ALIKE OR SOUND-ALIKE DRUG

RESEARCH ACTIVITY

1. Clark Kent calls to renew his Parkinson's disease medication. He does not remember the name of the drug. Review his patient profile, and make a list of the drugs for Parkinson's disease. Search the Internet to find pictures of the drugs, and then develop a list of questions you might ask to identify the drug he is requesting.

Last Name: Kent   First Name: Clark   Gender: M

Address: 1310 34th Ave. S #310   City: Anytown   DOB: 12-14-51

Allergies: NKA   Disc: Phone: 725-2743

Insurance: PCS Plan: 05   Group: 54873456   ID: 536234177   Copay: $7.00/$10

DATE	RX#	DRUG AND STRENGTH	MD	RF
11/7/06	236742	Sinemet 10-100 mg #90	Jones MD	2
12/05/06	236742	Sinemet 10-100 mg #90	Jones MD	1
1/4/07	236755	Sinemet 25-100 mg #90	Jones MD	0
1/4/07	236756	Phenytoin 100 mg #90	Jones MD	2
2/3/07	321477	Sinemet 25-100 mg CR #120	Jones MD	4
2/3/07	236756	Phenytoin 100 mg #90	Jones MD	1
3/2/07	321477	Sinemet 25-100 mg CR #120	Jones MD	3
3/26/07	344580	Demerol 100 mg #18	Bean DDS	0
3/26/07	344581	Amoxil 500 mg #9	Bean DDS	1
4/5/07	384222	Tegretol XR 300 mg #60	Jones MD	0
4/5/07	384223	benztropine 0.5 mg #30	Jones MD	0
5/13/07	384883	amitriptyline 10 mg #30	Jones MD	2
5/22/07	385129	Keppra 500 mg #60	Jones MD	1
5/22/07	385130	selegiline 5 mg #30	Jones MD	1

Make a list of the antiparkinson medications listed in his profile. (Give the brand and generic names.)

Make a list of questions you might ask to identify the current drug he is requesting.

ANTIPARKINSON DRUG	DRUG IDENTIFICATION QUESTIONS
	1.
	2.
	3.

9 Treatment of Seizure Disorders

TERMS AND DEFINITIONS

Match each term with the correct definition below. Some terms may not be used.

A. Anoxia

B. Aura

C. Convulsions

D. Epilepsy

E. Febrile seizure

F. Gingival hyperplasia

G. Hirsutism

H. Petit mal seizure

I. Seizure threshold

J. Simple focal seizures

K. Status epilepticus

L. Tonic-clonic (grand mal) seizure

M. Complex focal seizures

N. Eclampsia

O. Generalized seizures

P. Myoclonic seizure

1. The term that refers to a person's susceptibility to seizures is _____.

2. _____ is defined as a recurrent seizure disorder characterized by a sudden, excessive, disorderly discharge of cerebral neurons.

3. The term used to describe excessive growth of body hair (especially in women) is _____.

4. A _____ is associated with a sudden spike in body temperature.

5. _____ is a medical emergency brought on by repeated generalized seizures that can produce _____, a lack of oxygen to the brain.

6. _____ are generalized seizures that cause stiffening of the limbs, difficulty breathing, and jerking movements and are followed by limpness of the limbs and disorientation.

7. A _____ is characterized by a sudden contraction of muscles and is caused by seizures.

8. The term used to describe the condition in which gum tissue overgrows the teeth is _____.

9. An _____ is an unusual sensation or auditory, visual, or olfactory hallucination that is experienced just before the onset of a seizure.

10. _____, or absence seizure, is characterized by brief periods of unconsciousness and vacant stares.

11. _____ affect only one part of the brain and cause the person to experience unusual sensations or feelings.

12. _____ produces a blank stare, disorientation, repetitive actions, and memory loss.

13. _____ is a life-threatening condition that can develop in pregnant women.

14. _____ spreads across both cerebral hemispheres and includes tonic-clonic, myoclonic, and petit mal seizures.

15. A _____ is a seizure that is characterized by jerking muscle movements and is caused by contraction of the major muscle groups.

MULTIPLE CHOICE

1. Approximately _____ of the population has epilepsy.
   A. 1%
   B. 5%
   C. 10%
   D. 20%

2. Seizures may be caused by all of the following except _____.
   A. infection and high fevers
   B. anxiety and schizophrenia
   C. tumors and head trauma
   D. hypoglycemia and cerebrovascular disease
   E. drug and alcohol withdrawal

3. Sudden, excessive neuronal firing associated with seizures is inhibited by drugs that _____.
   A. inhibit dopamine synthesis and release
   B. delay the inflow of sodium ions and bind to T-type calcium channels
   C. inhibit serotonin reuptake
   D. inhibit acetylcholine

4. Which symptom is *not* associated with grand mal seizures? _____
   A. Convulsions
   B. Brief vacant stare
   C. Jerking movements
   D. Difficulty breathing

5. A grand mal seizure is also known as _____.
   A. a petit mal seizure
   B. a tonic-clonic seizure
   C. status epilepticus
   D. a febrile seizure

6. Joe Sherman is taking Lamictal 25-mg tablets. Which of the following warnings should he be given? _____
   A. MAY CAUSE DROWSINESS OR DIZZINESS
   B. AVOID ALCOHOL
   C. AVOID SUNLIGHT
   D. TAKE ON AN EMPTY STOMACH
   E. A and B

7. Which drug can be prescribed for seizures and

   neuropathic pain? _____
   A. Dilantin
   B. Neurontin
   C. Depakote
   D. Zarontin

8. June Schultz is taking Depakote 250-mg delayed-release tablets. Which of the following warnings should she be

   given? _____
   A. MAY CAUSE DROWSINESS OR DIZZINESS
   B. TAKE WITH FOOD
   C. SWALLOW WHOLE; DO NOT CRUSH OR CHEW
   D. AVOID ALCOHOL
   E. all of the above

9. Pharmacy technicians should dispense the same

   manufacturer's formulation of _____
   each time a prescription is filled, if possible.
   A. lamotrigene
   B. topiramate
   C. phenytoin
   D. levetiracetam

FILL IN THE BLANK: DRUG NAMES

1. What is the *generic name* for Dilantin? _____

2. What is the *generic name* for Depakote? _____

3. What is a *generic name* for Cerebyx? _____

4. What is the *generic name* for Depakene? _____

5. What is a *brand name* for carbamazepine? _____

6. What is a *brand name* for oxcarbazepine? _____

7. What is the *generic name* for Neurontin? _____

8. What is the *brand name* for tiagabine? _____

9. What is a *generic name* for Lyrica (United States)? _____

10. What is the *generic name* for Sabril (Canada)? _____

11. What is a *brand name* for ethosuximide? _____

12. What is the *brand name* for primidone? _____

13. What is the *brand name* for clonazepam? _____

14. What is the *generic name* for Lamictal? _____

15. What is a *brand name* for diazepam? _____

16. What is the *brand name* for levetiracetam? _____

17. What is the *generic name* for Topamax? _____

18. What is a *generic name* for Zonegran? _____

MATCHING

1. _____ Myoclonic seizure

2. _____ Complex focal seizure

3. _____ Generalized seizure

4. _____ Febrile seizure

5. _____ Petit mal seizure

A. Characterized by brief periods of unconsciousness and vacant stares

B. Associated with a sudden spike in body temperature

C. Associated with a blank stare, disorientation, repetitive actions, and memory loss

D. Seizures that spread across both cerebral hemispheres

E. Characterized by jerking muscle movements and caused by contraction of major muscle groups

MATCHING

Patient education is an essential component of therapeutics. Select the **best** warning label to apply to the prescription vial given to patients taking the drugs listed.

1. _____ Tegretol XR 200 mg

2. _____ Trileptal 300 mg/5 mL

3. _____ phenytoin 50-mg chewable tablets

4. _____ Neurontin 600 mg

A. AVOID ANTACIDS

B. TAKE WITH A GLASS OF WATER

C. SWALLOW WHOLE; DO NOT CRUSH OR CHEW

D. SHAKE WELL

E. AVOID ALCOHOL

MATCHING

Match each drug to its pharmacological classification.

1. _____ Tegretol 100 mg

2. _____ Depakene 250 mg/5 mL

3. _____ ethosuximide 250 mg/5 mL

4. _____ Neurontin 600 mg

5. _____ phenytoin 100 mg

A. hydantoins

B. valproates

C. iminostilbenes

D. GABA analogues

E. succinamides

TRUE OR FALSE

1. _____ Status epilepticus must be treated with intravenous medications.

2. _____ Nearly 75% of all seizures have no known cause.

3. _____ The aim of pharmaceutical treatment of seizures is to suppress seizure activity.

4. _____ Carbamazepine should be protected from light and moisture.

5. _____ Flashing or strobe lights, such as those used in fire alarm systems, can trigger a seizure in susceptible individuals with epilepsy.

6. _____ Depakote sprinkles must be swallowed whole.

CRITICAL THINKING

The following hard copies are brought to your pharmacy for filling. Identify the prescription error(s). (You already have the patient's full address on file.)

```
┌─────────────────────────────────────────┐
│        Micheal Vessalago, MD   Date _____ │
│            1221 Madison #310              │
│             Anytown, USA                  │
│  Pt. Name _____ Mary Smith _____ │
│  Address _____ │
│  Rx   Topamax 200mg                       │
│         1 BID                             │
│                                           │
│                                           │
│  Refills __11__                           │
│       Vessalago                           │
│  _____    _____ │
│  Substitution permitted   Dispense as written │
└─────────────────────────────────────────┘
```

1. Spot the error in the following

   prescription: _____
   A. Quantity missing
   B. Strength missing
   C. Strength incorrect
   D. Directions missing
   E. Dosage form incorrect

```
┌─────────────────────────────────────────┐
│        Anh Dang Tu, MD      Date _____    │
│            1145 Broadway                  │
│             Anytown, USA                  │
│  Pt. Name _____ Lili Ng _____ │
│  Address _____ │
│  Rx   phenytoin 10.0mg cap      #90       │
│         1 cap TID for epilepsy            │
│                                           │
│                                           │
│  Refills _____                           │
│              Tu                           │
│  _____    _____ │
│  Substitution permitted   Dispense as written │
└─────────────────────────────────────────┘
```

2. Spot the error in the following

   prescription: _____
   A. Quantity missing
   B. Directions incomplete
   C. Strength missing
   D. Strength incorrect
   E. Dosage form incorrect

```
┌─────────────────────────────────────────┐
│        Marc Cordova, MD     Date _____    │
│            1145 Broadway                  │
│             Anytown, USA                  │
│  Pt. Name _____ Sheila Wellcome _____ │
│  Address _____ │
│  Rx   Neurontin 600mg cap     #90         │
│         1 cap TID                         │
│                                           │
│                                           │
│  Refills _____                           │
│       Cordova                             │
│  _____    _____ │
│  Substitution permitted   Dispense as written │
└─────────────────────────────────────────┘
```

3. Spot the error in the following

   prescription: _____
   A. Quantity missing
   B. Directions incomplete
   C. Strength missing
   D. Strength incorrect
   E. Dosage form incorrect

4. List two pairs of drug names that have look-alike or sound-alike issues with drugs used to treat seizure disorders.

DRUG NAME	LOOK-ALIKE OR SOUND-ALIKE DRUG

5. Susan Heller has been diagnosed with epilepsy and prescribed Keppra, 500 mg 1 BID, increased by 500 mg per dose every 2 weeks, until she is taking 3 g daily. For approximately how many days will 200 tablets last? Please show your calculations.

_____

_____

_____

_____

_____

6. You receive a prescription from Sheila Harper for Trileptal to treat epilepsy. Sheila weighs 60 pounds. If Sheila should receive 9 mg/kg/day, approximately how many milligrams of Trileptal should she take every day? Please show your calculations.

_____

_____

_____

_____

_____

7. Adolescents treated for status epilepticus with lorazepam should receive 0.07 mg/kg/dose over 2 to 5 minutes (not more than 4 mg in a single dose); the dose may be repeated in 10 to 15 minutes. If Billy weighs 117 pounds, what dose should he be administered? Is this dose within the normal range? Please show your calculations.

_____

_____

_____

_____

_____

1. Research head injury and seizures at cdc.gov/ncipc/tbi/TBI.htm and epilepsyontario.org/client/EO/EOWeb.nsf/web/ BrainInjury. How can risks for head trauma be reduced?

_____

_____

_____

_____

_____

10 Treatment of Pain and Migraine Headache

TERMS AND DEFINITIONS

Match each term with the correct definition below. Some terms may not be used.

A. Acute pain

B. Acupuncture

C. Analgesic

D. Arthritis

E. Biofeedback

F. Chronic pain

G. Cyclo-oxygenase-2 inhibitor

H. Diabetic neuropathy

I. Dysphoria

J. Dynorphin

K. Endorphins

L. Enkephalins

M. Euphoria

N. Neuropathic pain

O. Nociceptors

P. Opioid

Q. Plasticity

R. Shingles

S. Substance P

T. Trigeminal neuralgia

U. Breakthrough pain

V. Cephalalgia

W. Cluster headache _____

X. Hyperalgesia _____

Y. Migraine _____

Z. NSAID _____

AA. Opiate naïve _____

BB. PCA _____

1. _____ are thin nerve fibers in skin, muscle, and other body tissues that carry pain signals.

2. _____ is a disorder that occurs in people with diabetes and causes numbness, pain, or tingling in the feet or legs.

3. A drug that reduces pain is called a(n) _____.

4. Naturally occuring or synthetically derived _____ analgesics have properties similar to those of morphine.

5. Sudden pain or _____ that results from injury or inflammation is usually self-limiting.

6. _____ is a procedure that involves the application of needles to precise points on the body.

7. Pain that persists for a long period of time that is worsened by psychological factors and is resistant to many medical treatments is classified as _____.

8. _____ is a condition that is associated with joint pain.

9. Painful skin rash associated with _____ is caused by the reactivation of the herpes zoster virus.

10. The peptide that is involved in the production of pain sensations and controls pain perception is called _____.

11. _____, _____, and _____ are natural painkillers.

12. _____ is a painful condition that produces intense, stabbing pain in areas of the face innervated by branches of the trigeminal nerve.

13. _____ is a feeling of emotional and/or mental discomfort, restlessness, and depression and is the opposite of _____.

14. _____ involves relaxation techniques and the gaining of self-control over muscle tension, heart rate, and skin temperature.

15. Analgesic, anti-inflammatory drugs that block the enzyme cyclo-oxygenase-2 are called _____.

16. The ability of the brain to restructure itself and adapt to injury is called _____.

17. A type of pain that is associated with nerve injury, called _____, may be caused by trauma, infection, or chronic diseases such as diabetes.

18. _____ is pain that occurs between scheduled doses of analgesics.

19. _____ is head pain.

20. _____ is intensely painful vascular headache that occurs in groups and produces pain on one side of the head.

21. _____ is heightened sensitivity to pain that can result from treatment of chronic pain with high-dose opioids.

22. _____ is a vascular headache that is often accompanied by nausea and visual disturbances.

23. _____ is the acronym for nonsteroidal anti-inflammatory drug.

24. _____ means no current exposure to opioids.

25. _____ is patient-controlled analgesia.

MULTIPLE CHOICE

1. Duragesic patches should be replaced every

   _____ hours.
   A. 12
   B. 24
   C. 36
   D. 72

2. Buprenorphine tablets _____.
   A. may be prescribed by any licensed prescriber
   B. may only be prescribed for the treatment of opioid dependence by specially licensed and authorized prescribers
   C. are available in combination with naltrexone by the trade name Suboxone (United States)
   D. may cause excitation

3. If a patient has received too much Sublimaze in the operating room, which narcotic antagonist should be available to reverse respiratory depression?

   _____
   A. dipehnoxylate atropine
   B. naltrexone
   C. acetaminophen with codeine no. 4
   D. naloxone

4. Jenny, age 13, suffered a burn to 25% of her body. To ease the pain, her physician prescribed morphine

   sulfate. This drug is derived from _____.
   A. coca leaves
   B. opium poppy
   C. amphetamines
   D. codeine
   E. marijuana

5. Opioids differ from opiates because

   _____.
   A. opioids are narcotics
   B. opioids may be derived from natural or synthetic sources
   C. only opioids are controlled substances
   D. opioids are less potent than opiates

6. Which of the following two agents might be used to

   treat opioid-dependent patients? _____
   A. fentanyl and naltrexone
   B. methadone and hydrocodone
   C. Stadol and oxycodone
   D. Suboxone and naltrexone

7. Melissa Block has been given a prescription for Tylenol No. 3 following a tooth extraction. Which warning label would *not* be appropriate to place on

   her prescription vial? _____
   A. TAKE WITH FOOD
   B. MAY CAUSE DROWSINESS; ALCOHOL MAY INTENSIFY THIS EFFECT
   C. AVOID PROLONGED EXPOSURE TO SUNLIGHT
   D. MAY BE HABIT FORMING
   E. AVOID OPERATION OF HAZARDOUS MACHINERY

8. Many pain medications contain opioid plus acetaminophen. What is the maximum adult dose

   of acetaminophen per day? _____
   A. 1 g
   B. 2 g
   C. 3 g
   D. 4 g

9. Which of these drugs is an opioid antagonist?

_____

A. oxycodone
B. Vicodin
C. Revia
D. Dolophine

10. Which of the following medicines is classified as a mixed opioid agonist/antagonist?

_____

A. Revia
B. Tylox
C. Demerol
D. Stadol nasal spray

FILL IN THE BLANK: DRUG NAMES

1. What is the **brand name** for hydrocodone and ibuprofen? _____

2. What is the **generic name** for Tylenol with Codeine No. 4? _____

3. What is a **brand name** for hydromorphone? _____

4. What is the **generic name** for Actiq and Duragesic? _____

5. What is the **brand name** for meperidine? _____

6. What is the **generic name** for Vicodin (United States)? _____

7. What are **brand name**s for methadone? _____ and

_____

8. What are **brand name**s for sustained-release morphine? _____ and

_____

9. What is a **brand name** for sustained-release oxycodone? _____

10. What is the **generic name** for Percocet? _____

11. What is the **generic name** for Numorphan? _____

12. What is a **brand name** for buprenorphine? _____

13. What is the **brand name** for naloxone? _____

14. What is the **generic name** for Stadol? _____

15. What is the **brand name** for naltrexone? _____

MATCHING

Patient education is an essential component of therapeutics. Select the **best** warning label to apply to the prescription vial given to patients taking the drugs listed.

1. _____ flurbiprofen 100 mg   A. ROTATE SITE OF APPLICATION

2. _____ Oxycontin 30 mg   B. SWALLOW WHOLE; DO NOT CRUSH OR CHEW

3. _____ Duragesic 50 μg   C. AVOID ASPIRIN AND RELATED DRUGS

MATCHING

Match each drug to its pharmacological classification.

1. _____ Duragesic   A. Opioid agonist

2. _____ Stadol   B. Opioid mixed agonist

3. _____ Narcan   C. Opioid antagonist

4. _____ Lodine   D. NSAID

TRUE OR FALSE

1. _____ Opiate naïve means without knowledge or understanding of the use of painkillers.

2. _____ Duragesic patches should be dispensed with instructions on proper storage and disposal to prevent accidental poisoning.

3. _____ Patient-controlled analgesia increases the risk for drug dependency.

4. _____ Patient-controlled analgesia permits patients to control the frequency of administration of their dose of pain medications.

5. _____ Endorphins, enkephalins, and dynorphin are substances that are released by the body in response to painful stimuli and act as natural painkillers.

6. _____ Biofeedback and acupuncture are nonpharmacological treatments for pain.

7. _____ The peptide that is involved in the production of pain sensations and controls pain perception is called substance X.

8. _____ Celebrex is the only remaining COX-2 inhibitor marketed in the United States and Canada.

CRITICAL THINKING

The following hard copies are brought to your pharmacy for filling. Identify the prescription error(s). (You already have the patient's full address on file.)

| Kathy Principi, MD   Date _____ |
| 1145 Broadway |
| Anytown, USA |

Pt. Name _____ Sheila Wilcox _____

Address _____

℞   *Duragesic 25mcg*   *#5*
     1 patch daily

Refills _____

____*Principi*____   _____
Substitution permitted   Dispense as written

1. Spot the error in the following prescription:

   _____

   A. Quantity missing
   B. Strength missing
   C. Strength incorrect
   D. Directions incorrect
   E. Dosage form incorrect

```
          Kathy Principi, MD      Date _____
             1145 Broadway
             Anytown, USA

Pt. Name _____ Ellen Wilber _____
Address _____
R   Stadol 10mg/ml    1 bottle
     1 spray in each nostril repeat when needed


Refills _____
____ Principi _____    _____
Substitution permitted        Dispense as written
```

2. Spot the error in the following prescription:

   _____

   A. Quantity missing
   B. Directions incorrect
   C. Strength missing
   D. Strength incorrect
   E. Dosage form incorrect

```
          Marc Cordova, MD       Date _____
             1145 Broadway
             Anytown, USA

Pt. Name _____ Alvin Sorrento _____
Address _____
R   hydrocodone 5mg/acetaminophen 500mg tab
     i tab q 4-6h


Refills _____
____ Cordova _____    _____
Substitution permitted        Dispense as written
```

3. Spot the error in the following prescription:

   _____

   A. Quantity missing
   B. Strength missing
   C. Strength incorrect
   D. Directions incorrect
   E. Dosage form incorrect

4. List four pairs of drug names that have look-alike or sound-alike issues with drugs used to treat pain.

DRUG NAME	LOOK-ALIKE OR SOUND-ALIKE DRUG

5. Nick Harper has been prescribed a pain "cocktail" containing Dolophine, 10 mg/5 mL, and hydroxyzine HCl, 50 mg/5 mL, in cherry syrup. He is instructed to take one teaspoonful every 6 hours. How many Dolophine tablets must you use to prepare 150 mL of the pain cocktail? (You will be using Dolophine 5-mg tablets.) Please show your calculations.

_____

_____

_____

_____

_____

_____

6. If Mr. Strong is admitted to the hospital and administered Buprenex, how much will you draw up in the syringe for a 0.6-mg dose? How many milliliters (mL) will be needed per day if the dosage range is 0.3 to 0.6 mg every 6 hours? (Buprenex 0.3 mg/mL.) Please show your calculations.

_____

_____

_____

_____

_____

RESEARCH ACTIVITY

1. The fear of prescribing, dispensing, or taking opioid pain medications is called *opiophobia*. Use the Internet to research controlled substances. Locate treatment guidelines for terminal illness. When are concerns warranted? When are concerns not warranted?

_____

_____

_____

_____

_____

11 Treatment of Alzheimer's Disease

TERMS AND DEFINITIONS

Match each term with the correct definition below. Some terms may not be used.

A. Acetylcholinesterase

B. Alzheimer's disease

C. Dementia

D. Neurodegeneration

E. Neuroprotective

F. Plaques

G. Tangles

H. *ApoE4* allele

1. The enzyme that degrades the neurotransmitter acetylcholine is called _____.

2. The term used to describe the condition associated with a loss of memory and cognition is _____.

3. A drug that is _____ protects nerve cells from damage.

4. Twisted fibers made up of clumps of protein are called _____ and can interfere with nerve signal transmission.

5. _____ is defined as destruction of nerve cells.

6. _____ is a neurodegenerative disease that causes memory loss, behavioral changes, and immobility.

7. Sticky, dense beta-amyloid–filled spaces between neurons called _____ interfere with the transmission of signals between neurons.

8. _____ is a defective form of apoliprotein E that is associated with Alzheimer's disease.

MULTIPLE CHOICE

1. Abnormal structures called plaques and tangles that form in persons with Alzheimer's disease

    _____.
    A. increase transmission of messages between neurons
    B. decrease transmission of messages between neurons
    C. have no effect on transmission of messages between neurons

2. Which drug used for the treatment of Alzheimer's disease is a glutamate inhibitor? _____
    A. tacrine (Cognex)
    B. donepezil (Aricept)
    C. rivastigmine (Exelon)
    D. galantamine (Reminyl)
    E. memantine (Namenda)

3. A defective form of apolipoprotein E that is associated with Alzheimer's disease is _____.
    A. *ApoE2* allele
    B. *ApoE4* allele
    C. *ApoE6* allele
    D. *ApoE8* allele

4. Rivastigmine premixed solution must be used within _____ hours of mixing.
    A. 2
    B. 4
    C. 6
    D. 8

5. Alzheimer's disease is a neurodegenerative disease that results in _____.
    A. excess muscle movement
    B. tremors
    C. memory loss
    D. headache

6. Select the pair of neurotransmitters that are involved in Alzheimer's disease. _____
    A. Acetylcholine and glutamate
    B. Acetylcholine and norepinephrine
    C. Norepinephrine and histamine
    D. Norepinephrine and serotonin

FILL IN THE BLANK: DRUG NAMES

1. What is the ***brand name*** for donepezil? _____

2. What is the ***brand name*** for rivastigmine? _____

3. What is the ***generic name*** for Namenda? _____

4. What is the ***brand name*** for galantamine? _____

MATCHING

Patient education is an essential component of therapeutics. Select the **best** warning label to apply to the prescription vial given to patients taking the drugs listed.

1. _____ donepezil   A. MAY CAUSE DIZZINESS OR DROWSINESS

2. _____ memantine   B. TAKE WITH FOOD

3. _____ galantamine ER   C. DISSOLVE IN MOUTH

4. _____ rivastigmine   D. SWALLOW WHOLE; DO NOT CRUSH OR CHEW

TRUE OR FALSE

1. _____ Plaques are dense substances composed of a protein called beta-amyloid.

2. _____ Tangles are twisted strands of nerves that may cause Alzhemier's disease.

3. _____ Neurodegeneration is the destruction of nerve cells.

4. _____ Dementia is a normal part of the aging process.

5. _____ There are four classes of glutamatergic receptors.

CRITICAL THINKING

The following hard copies are brought to your pharmacy for filling. Identify the prescription error(s). (You already have the patient's full address on file.)

```
┌─────────────────────────────────────────────────┐
│          Kathy Principi, MD      Date _____    │
│          1145 Broadway                           │
│          Anytown, USA                            │
│                                                  │
│  Pt. Name _____ Ellen Wilber _____  │
│  Address _____│
│  ℞   Imitrex 10mg     1 bottle                   │
│        1 spray in each nostril                   │
│                                                  │
│                                                  │
│  Refills _____                                  │
│  ____Principi_____    _____  │
│  Substitution permitted   Dispense as written    │
└─────────────────────────────────────────────────┘
```

1. Spot the error in the following prescription:

   _____

   A. Quantity missing
   B. Directions incomplete
   C. Strength missing
   D. Strength incorrect
   E. Dosage form incorrect

2. List four pairs of drug names that have look-alike or sound-alike issues with drugs used to treat migraine headache and those used to treat Alzheimer's disease.

DRUG NAME	LOOK-ALIKE OR SOUND-ALIKE DRUG

12 Treatment of Sleep Disorders and Attention-Deficit Hyperactivity Disorder

TERMS AND DEFINITIONS

Match each term with the correct definition below. Some terms may not be used.

A. Circadian rhythm

B. Depressant

C. Disinhibition

D. Hypnotic

E. Insomnia

F. Melatonin

G. Non–rapid eye movement sleep

H. Rapid eye movement sleep

I. Rebound hypersomnia

J. Sedative

K. Stimulants

L. Sympathomimetic

1. _____ is a hormone released by the pineal gland that makes a person feel drowsy.

2. A drug that decreases activity in the brain is called a _____ and is used as a sedative or hypnotic to promote drowsiness and relaxation.

3. _____, or excessive sleep, is an adverse effect associated with long-term use of drugs that depress rapid eye movement and non–rapid eye movement sleep.

4. Drugs that increase activity in the brain are called _____ and can be used to treat attention-deficit/hyperactivity disorder (ADHD) and narcolepsy.

5. A _____ is a drug that is used to treat _____, a condition characterized by difficulty falling asleep and/or staying asleep.

6. The stages of sleep are categorized as _____ and _____.

7. One adverse effect of barbiturates is _____, the opposite of inhibition.

8. A _____ is a drug whose effects mimic the effects produced by stimulation of the sympathetic nervous system.

9. The term used to describe biological change that occurs according to time cycles is _____.

10. A _____ is a drug that causes relaxation and promotes drowsiness.

MULTIPLE CHOICE

1. Sleep deprivation is linked to all of the following

   except _____.
   A. increased illness
   B. motor vehicle accidents
   C. increased mental agility
   D. lack of productivity

2. The pineal gland controls the release of

   _____, a hormone that makes people
   feel drowsy.
   A. cortisol
   B. thyroid hormone
   C. estrogen
   D. testosterone
   E. melatonin

3. Which of the following is *not* linked to insomnia?

   _____
   A. Sleep apnea
   B. Use of depressant drugs
   C. Consumption of caffeinated beverages and foods
   D. Use of stimulant drugs
   E. Chronic pain and illness

4. Select the advice that would *not* be a tip to prevent

   insomnia. _____
   A. Avoid stimulants close to bedtime.
   B. Adopt a regular sleeping schedule.
   C. Take daytime naps.
   D. Exercise.
   E. Do not lie in bed awake.

5. Prescription drugs used to treat insomnia are

   _____.
   A. barbiturates and benzodiazepines
   B. decongestants and analgesics
   C. NSAIDs and antibiotics
   D. barbiturates and decongestants

6. Homer Street calls the pharmacy to renew his
   "sleeping pill." His profile shows he has recently
   taken the drugs listed below. Which drug is the

   "sleeping pill"? _____
   A. Buspirone
   B. Alprazolam
   C. Triazolam
   D. Fluoxetine

7. The pharmacist reminds Mr. Street to avoid concur-

   rent use of _____ when he takes his
   "sleeping pill."
   A. ASA
   B. antacids
   C. APAP
   D. alcohol

8. Pharmaceutical treatment of ADHD is achieved
   with the administration of all of the following

   except _____.
   A. temazepam
   B. methylphenidate
   C. Adderall
   D. Concerta

9. Which warning label should *not* be applied to
   prescriptions filled for modafinil?

   _____.
   A. AVOID ALCOHOL
   B. MAY DECREASE EFFECT OF ORAL
   CONTRACEPTIVES
   C. MAY CAUSE DROWSINESS
   D. MAY BE HABIT FORMING

10. Which warning label should *not* be affixed to
    prescription vials for Adderall XR?

    _____
    A. TAKE WITH FOOD
    B. MAY BE HABIT FORMING
    C. SWALLOW WHOLE; DO NOT CRUSH
    OR CHEW
    D. MAY CAUSE DROWSINESS

FILL IN THE BLANK: DRUG NAMES

1. What is the *brand name* for amobarbital? _____

2. What is the *generic name* for Nembutal? _____

3. What is a *brand name* for secobarbital? _____

4. What is the *generic name* for Dalmane? _____

5. What is the *generic name* for Restoril? _____

6. What is the *generic name* for Halcion? _____

7. What is the *generic name* for Lunesta (United States)? _____

8. What is the *generic name* for Sonata (United States) and Starnoc (Canada)? _____

9. What is the *generic name* for Ambien (United States)? _____

10. What is the *generic name* for Imovane (Canada)? _____

11. What is the *brand name* for amphetamine plus dextroamphetamine? _____

12. What is the *generic name* for Provigil (United States)? _____

13. What is the *brand name* for dextroamphetamine? _____

14. What are *brand names* for methylphenidate? _____

15. What is the *brand name* for atomoxetine? _____

MATCHING

Match each drug to its pharmacological classification.

1. _____ Strattera

2. _____ Concerta

3. _____ Halcion

4. _____ Seconal

A. barbiturate

B. benzodiazepine

C. amphetamine

D. nonamphetamine stimulant

TRUE OR FALSE

1. _____ Rapid eye movement sleep is the stage of sleep where dreaming occurs.

2. _____ Pharmacological treatment for insomnia is recommended for long-term therapy.

3. _____ Our normal sleep–wake cycle is linked to changes in sunlight.

4. _____ Melatonin and valerian root are natural remedies that have proven effectiveness for promoting sleep.

5. _____ Increased appetite is an adverse effect associated with the administration of amphetamines.

6. _____ Concerta should be taken in the morning to avoid insomnia.

The following hard copies are brought to your pharmacy for filling. Identify the prescription error(s). (You already have the patient's full address on file.)

| Micheal Vessalago, MD   Date _____ |
| 1221 Madison #310 |
| Anytown, USA |

Pt. Name _____ Bart Klitgaard _____

Address _____

℞ secobarbital 100mg caps   #10

  i HS

Refills 2

Vessalago   AV1111119   _____

Substitution permitted   Dispense as written

1. Spot the error in the following prescription:

   _____

   A. Quantity missing
   B. RF limit exceeded
   C. Strength missing
   D. Strength incorrect
   E. Dosage form incorrect

| Marc Cordova, MD   Date _____ |
| 1145 Broadway |
| Anytown, USA |

Pt. Name _____ Crystal Boelle _____

Address _____

℞ triazolam 0.25mg

  i tab at bedtime

Refills _____

_____   *Cordova*   _____

Substitution permitted   Dispense as written

2. Spot the error in the following prescription:

   _____

   A. Quantity missing
   B. RF limit exceeded
   C. Strength missing
   D. Strength incorrect
   E. Dosage form incorrect

3. List two pairs of drug names that have look-alike or sound-alike issues with drugs used to treat sleep disorders and those used to treat ADHD.

DRUG NAME	LOOK-ALIKE OR SOUND-ALIKE DRUG

1. Controversy exists with regard to the increasing numbers of diagnoses for ADHD and treatment for this disorder with stimulants. Do research on ADHD, and give reasons for and against treatment of it. Access the National Library of Medicine website (nlm.nih.gov/medlineplus/attentiondeficithyperactivitydisorder.html) or other websites to complete the research activity.

_____

_____

_____

_____

_____

13 Neuromuscular Blockade

TERMS AND DEFINITIONS

Match each term with the correct definition below. Some terms may not be used.

A. Anaphylactic shock

B. Blepharoptosis

C. Botulinum toxin

D. Central-acting muscle relaxants

E. Depolarizing neuromuscular blockers

F. Diaphoresis (hyperhidrosis)

G. End plate

H. Endotracheal intubation

I. Neuromuscular junction

J. Nondepolarizing competitive blockers

K. Peripheral-acting muscle relaxants

L. Sole plate

M. Tetanus

N. Acetylcholinesterase

1. The space between the motor neuron end plate and the muscle sole plate that neurotransmitters must cross is called the _____.

2. _____ is the process of inserting a tube down into the trachea, or windpipe, to facilitate mechanical ventilation.

3. _____ is a condition that causes eyelid muscles to droop.

4. Drugs that compete with acetylcholine for binding sites are called _____.

5. The medical term for excessive sweating is _____.

6. A projection extending off the end of a motor neuron is called an _____ and is where the neurotransmitter acetylcholine is released.

7. _____ block nerve transmission between the motor end plate and skeletal muscle receptors.

8. The portion of the membrane of muscle cells that receives messages transmitted by motor neurons is called

the _____.

9. The fatal condition _____ is characterized by continuous muscle spasm and is also known as "lockjaw."

10. Drugs that produce relaxation of muscles by central nervous system depression, blocking nerve transmission

between the spinal cord and muscles, are called _____.

11. A poison produced by the bacterium *Clostridium botulinum*, _____, causes muscle paralysis.

12. _____ is an acute, life-threatening allergic reaction.

13. _____ produce sustained depolarization by causing acetylcholine receptor sites to convert to an inactive state.

14. An enzyme that degrades acetlycholine and reverses acetylcholine-induced depolarization is called

_____.

MULTIPLE CHOICE

1. Depolarizing neuromuscular blockers produce sustained depolarization by causing _____ receptor sites to convert to an inactive state.
   A. norepinephrine
   B. dopamine
   C. GABA
   D. acetylcholine

2. Which symptom is *not* associated with anaphylactic shock? _____
   A. Peripheral vasodilation
   B. Bradycardia
   C. Bronchospasm
   D. Laryngeal edema
   E. Airway obstruction

3. Botox injections are made from a substance derived from botulinum toxin that works by

   _____.
   A. preventing reuptake of norepinephrine
   B. preventing reuptake of serotonin
   C. preventing nerve impulses from reaching the muscle
   D. increasing nerve impulses to muscle

4. Neuromuscular blocking drugs are classified as

   "_____" by the Interdisciplinary Safe Medication Use Expert Committee of the United States Pharmacopoeia.
   A. dangerous
   B. high alert
   C. low alert
   D. use with caution

5. Select the drug that reverses the effects of neuromuscular blocking agents. _____
   A. vecuronium
   B. rocuronium
   C. neostigmine
   D. mivacurium
   E. pancuronium

6. Which problem associated with neuromuscular blocking drugs is *not* attributed to the dispensing

   pharmacy? _____
   A. Improper product selection
   B. Improper storage conditions
   C. Inappropriate dosing
   D. Improper labeling
   E. Inadequate patient monitoring

7. According to the Interdisciplinary Safe Medication Use Expert Committee of the United States Pharmacopoeia, the warning label _____ should always be placed on dispensed neuromuscular blocking drugs.
   A. KEEP IN REFRIGERATOR
   B. WARNING: PARALYZING AGENT (USE REQUIRES MECHANICAL VENTILATORY ASSISTANCE)
   C. WARNING: ALLERGIC REACTIONS POSSIBLE
   D. FOR ONE TIME USE ONLY

8. The onset of action of neuromuscular blocking drugs is rapid (1 to 4 minutes), and the duration of action

   _____.
   A. short (10 to 90 minutes)
   B. intermediate (1.5 to 3 hours)
   C. long (3 to 6 hours)

9. Botox injections can cause all of the following

   adverse reactions *except* _____.
   A. droopy eyelid muscles
   B. headache
   C. muscle weakness
   D. drowsiness
   E. flulike syndrome

10. Select the drug that does *not* decrease acetylcholine

   release. _____
   A. Donepezil
   B. Botulinum toxin
   C. Magnesium
   D. High doses of ethanol

FILL IN THE BLANK: DRUG NAMES

1. What is the *brand name* for succinylcholine? _____

2. What is the *generic name* for Botox? _____

3. What is the *generic name* for Nimbex? _____

4. What is the *brand name* for mivacurium? _____

5. What are *brand names* for rocuronium? _____

6. What is the *brand name* for vecuronium? _____

7. What is the *generic name* for Pavulon (Canada)? _____

8. What is the *brand name* for neostigmine? _____

TRUE OR FALSE

1. _____ Acetylcholinesterase is an enzyme that reverses acetylcholine-induced depolarization by degrading acetylcholine.

2. _____ Acetylcholine that is released from the nerve end plate binds to adrenergic receptor sites located in the muscle sole plate.

3. _____ Another name for diaphoresis is hypohidrosis.

4. _____ The endings *-curonium* and *-curium* are commonly used for nondepolarizing neuromuscular blockers.

5. _____ Look-alike packaging is a problem that can be attributed to drug manufacturers as well as to pharmacies dispensing drugs.

CRITICAL THINKING

1. List two pairs of drug names that have look-alike or sound-alike issues with drugs used for neuromuscular blockade.

DRUG NAME	LOOK-ALIKE OR SOUND-ALIKE DRUG

RESEARCH ACTIVITY

1. What causes tetanus, and how is the disorder managed? Check the *Merck Manual* website (merck.com/mmpe/index/ind_ne.html) and other websites to complete the research activity.

_____

_____

_____

_____

_____

14 Treatment of Muscle Spasms

TERMS AND DEFINITIONS

Match each term with the correct definition below. Some terms may not be used.

A. Amyotrophic lateral sclerosis

B. Cerebral palsy

C. Clonus

D. Lower motor neurons

E. Multiple sclerosis

F. Negative symptoms

G. Phenylketonuria

H. Positive symptoms

I. Sarcomere

J. Spasticity

K. Upper motor neurons

1. Persons who have _____ are unable to metabolize the amino acid phenylalanine to tyrosine.

2. _____ is a motor disorder that causes increased muscle tone, exaggerated tendon jerks, and hyperexcitable muscles.

3. Spasticity symptoms that can produce muscle weakness, decreased endurance, and reduction in the ability to make voluntary muscle movements are called _____.

4. _____ branch out from the spinal cord to the muscles and tissues of the body.

5. _____ is a neurological disorder that affects muscle movement and coordination.

6. Spasticity symptoms that cause muscle spasms and hyperexcitable reflexes are called _____.

7. Neurons that carry messages from the brain down to the spinal cord are called _____.

8. _____ is an autoimmune disease that causes progressive damage to nerves, resulting in spasticity, pain, mood changes, and other physical symptoms.

9. Involuntary rhythmic muscle contraction, called _____, causes the feet and wrists to involuntarily flex and relax.

10. _____ is also known as Lou Gehrig's disease.

11. The _____ is the contracting unit of muscle fibers.

MULTIPLE CHOICE

1. Select the condition that is a degenerative disease that causes muscle wasting and weakness.

   _____
   A. Amyotrophic lateral sclerosis (ALS)
   B. Huntington's disease
   C. Muscular sclerosis
   D. Parkinson's disease

2. Neurons that branch out from the spinal cord to the muscles and tissues of the body are called

   _____.
   A. upper motor neurons
   B. terminal neurons
   C. interneurons
   D. lower motor neurons

3. Botulnium toxins type A and B are used for the

   treatment of _____ and cervical
   dystonia.
   A. blepharospasms
   B. cerebral palsy
   C. spinal cord injury
   D. stroke spasticity

4. Nonpharmacological management of spasticity includes

   all of the following *except* _____.
   A. transcutaneous electrical stimulation (TENS)
   B. hot packs (thermal therapy)
   C. cold packs (cryotherapy)
   D. biofeedback
   E. physical therapy

5. Which drug is used for the treatment of muscle

   strain? _____
   A. carisoprodol
   B. diazepam
   C. dantrolene
   D. baclofen

6. Which of the muscle relaxants listed can discolor

   urine? _____
   A. diazepam
   B. chlorzoxazone
   C. methocarbamol
   D. B and C

7. Which medical condition is *not* associated with

   spasticity? _____
   A. Stroke
   B. Depression
   C. Spinal cord injury
   D. Cerebral palsy
   E. Head injury

8. Select the **true** statement. _____
   A. Spasticity may be due to a decrease in neu-rotransmitters that carry excitatory messages.
   B. The development of loose and flexible muscles is the final phase in the development of spasticity.
   C. After a spinal cord injury, spasticity develops because the body grows new synapses, resulting in a stronger reflex response.
   D. Decreased muscle tone is one of the phases in the development of spasticity.

9. Peripherally acting skeletal muscle relaxants act at

   the _____.
   A. brain
   B. spinal cord
   C. neuromuscular junction
   D. limbs

10. Select the peripherally acting skeletal muscle

    relaxant. _____
    A. chlorzoxazone
    B. cyclobenzaprine
    C. dantrolene
    D. methocarbamol
    E. tizanidine

FILL IN THE BLANK: DRUG NAMES

1. What is a *brand name* for diazepam? _____

2. What is the *generic name* for Dantrium? _____

3. What is a *brand name* for baclofen? _____

4. What is the *generic name* for Zanaflex? _____

5. What is the *brand name* for chlorzoxazone? _____

6. What is a *brand name* for methocarbamol? _____

7. What is the *brand name* for orphenadrine? _____

8. What is the *generic name* for Soma (United States)? _____

9. What is the *generic name* for Robaxisal (United States) and Extra-Strength Muscle and Back Pain Relief (Canada)?

   _____

MATCHING

Patient education is an essential component of therapeutics. Select the **best** warning label to apply to the prescription vial given to patients taking the drugs listed.

1. _____ orphenadrine extended release

2. _____ diazepam 10 mg

3. _____ methocarbamol 500 mg

4. _____ baclofen 10 mg

A. MAY DISCOLOR URINE

B. TAKE WITH FOOD

C. MAY BE HABIT FORMING

D. SWALLOW WHOLE; DO NOT CRUSH OR CHEW

TRUE OR FALSE

1. _____ The myelin sheath around neurons acts as an electrical conductor and slows the velocity of impulse transmission.

2. _____ Skeletal muscle relaxants should be used along with nonpharmaceutical therapies such as rest, exercise, cryotherapy, and physical therapy.

3. _____ There are five phases in the development of spasticity.

4. _____ Drugs used in the treatment of spasticity are classified as centrally acting and peripherally acting drugs.

5. _____ Baclofen is a centrally acting drug that looks and acts like 5-hydroxytryptamine (5-HT), a naturally occurring neurotransmitter.

CRITICAL THINKING

The following hard copies are brought to your pharmacy for filling. Identify the prescription error(s). (You already have the patient's full address on file.)

Kathy Principi, MD Date _____
1145 Broadway
Anytown, USA
 	
Pt. Name _____ Sheila Wilcox _____
Address _____
 	
℞ methocarbamol #30
    i tab QID
 	
Refills _____
   Principi
_____   _____
Substitution permitted   Dispense as written
	1. Spot the error in the following prescription:
	
	_____
	
	A. Quantity missing
	B. Strength missing
	C. Strength incorrect
	D. Directions incorrect
	E. Dosage form incorrect

Kathy Principi, MD Date _____
1145 Broadway
Anytown, USA
 	
Pt. Name _____ Ellen Wilber _____
Address _____
 	
℞ Zanaflex #30
    1-2 tablets TID
 	
Refills _____
   Principi
_____   _____
Substitution permitted   Dispense as written
	2. Spot the error in the following prescription:
	
	_____
	
	A. Quantity missing
	B. Directions incorrect
	C. Strength missing
	D. Strength incorrect
	E. Dosage form incorrect

Marc Cordova, MD Date _____ 1145 Broadway Seattle, WA 98122 Pt. Name _____ Alvin Sorrento _____ Address _____ ℞ Lioresal 5mg TID Refills _____ Cordova _____ _____ Substitution permitted Dispense as written	3. Spot the error in the following prescription: _____ A. Quantity missing B. Dose is excessive C. Strength missing D. Strength incorrect

4. List four pairs of drug names that have look-alike or sound-alike issues with drugs used to treat muscle spasms.

DRUG NAME	LOOK-ALIKE OR SOUND-ALIKE DRUG

RESEARCH ACTIVITY

The use of botulinum toxin for the treatment of spasticity is unlabeled. Conduct an Internet search on the off-label or unapproved use of medicines, and then answer the following questions.

1. Is off-label use legal?

_____

_____

_____

_____

_____

2. When might it be appropriate?

_____

_____

_____

_____

_____

_____

15 Treatment of Autoimmune Diseases That Affect the Musculoskeletal System

TERMS AND DEFINITIONS

Match each term with the correct definition below. Some terms may not be used.

A. Antinuclear antibody

B. Autoimmune disease

C. Autoantibody

D. Demyelination

E. Interferons

F. Multiple sclerosis

G. Myasthenia gravis

H. Myelin

 I. Myelin basic protein

J. Myositis

K. Plaques

L. Rheumatoid arthritis

M. Rheumatoid factor

N. Synovium

O. Systemic lupus erythematosus

P. Tumor necrosis factor

Q. Ataxia

R. Polymyositis

1. _____ enhance T-cell recognition of antigens and produce immune system suppression.

2. The fatty covering insulating nerve cells in the brain and spinal cord is called _____.

3. _____ is an autoimmune disease that causes chronic inflammation of the muscles.

4. Damage caused by recurrent inflammation of myelin, for example, _____, results in nervous system scars that interrupt communication between the nerves and the rest of the body.

5. The immunoglobulin (antibody) _____ is present in many people who have _____, a chronic disease characterized by inflammation of the joints.

6. A disease that occurs when the immune system turns against the parts of the body it is designed to protect is called an _____.

7. The inflammatory cytokine _____ is found in the synovial fluid of people with rheumatoid arthritis.

8. A major component of myelin, _____ can be detected in the cerebrospinal fluid of people with multiple sclerosis.

9. _____ is an abnormal antibody that attacks the nucleus of normal cells in the body.

10. _____ is an autoimmune disease that affects nearly all body systems.

11. _____ is an autoimmune disease in which muscle cells are attacked at the neuromuscular junction, causing muscle weakness.

12. The _____ is a thin layer of tissue that lines the joint space.

13. _____ are patchy areas of inflammation and demyelination that disrupt nerve signals between the brain and the rest of the body.

14. _____ is an autoimmune disease that causes progressive damage to nerves, resulting in spasticity, pain, and other physical symptoms and mood changes.

15. The term used to describe an abnormal antibody that attacks healthy cells and tissues is _____.

16. _____ refers to a condition in which the muscles fail to function in a coordinated manner.

17. _____ is a form of myositis that affects multiple muscles, mainly muscles closest to the trunk.

MULTIPLE CHOICE

1. Which autoimmune disease affects nearly all body systems? _____
   A. Myasthenia gravis
   B. Myositis
   C. Rheumatoid arthritis
   D. Systemic lupus erythematosus
   E. Multiple sclerosis

2. Select the warning label that should *not* be applied to prescriptions for cyclosporine oral solution. _____
   A. DO NOT REFRIGERATE
   B. PROTECT FROM LIGHT
   C. PREPARE INJECTIONS IN GLASS
   D. REFRIGERATE; DO NOT FREEZE

3. Cyclosporine parenteral solution is stable for _____ hours in normal saline glass bottles.
   A. 6
   B. 9
   C. 12
   D. 24

4. Select the drug that must be disposed of in the cytotoxic waste containers (including intravenous bags, sets, and tubing and gloves). _____
   A. mitoxantrone
   B. methylprednisolone
   C. sulfasalazine
   D. Arava

5. Select the autoimmune disorder that does *not* affect the muscles. _____
   A. Myasthenia gravis
   B. Graves' disease
   C. Multiple sclerosis
   D. Rheumatoid arthritis
   E. Systemic lupus erythematosus

6. Which is *not* a treatment goal of current drug therapy for autoimmune disease affecting the musculoskeletal system? _____
   A. Suppressing inflammation
   B. Suppressing pain
   C. Suppressing the immune system response
   D. Cure

7. Select the **true** statement. _____
   A. Biological response modifiers stimulate the release of cells that mobilize to fight what the body believes is a harmful invasion.
   B. Biological response modifiers interfere with the activity of cytokines, leukocytes, B cells, and T cells.
   C. Selective COX-2 inhibitors decrease the risk for cardiovascular toxicity and gastrointestinal ulceration.
   D. Tumor necrosis factor-alpha inhibitors are produced by the body and block the inflammatory process.

8. Gold compounds are used in the treatment of

   _____.
   A. rheumatoid arthritis
   B. multiple sclerosis
   C. myositis
   D. systemic lupus erythematosus

9. Which drug is used for the treatment of multiple

   sclerosis? _____
   A. auranofin
   B. interferon-beta-1b
   C. sulfasalazine
   D. infliximab
   E. cyclosporine

10. Which drug is *not* used for the treatment of rheumatoid arthritis?
   A. Remicade
   B. gold salts
   C. leflunomide
   D. dantrolene
   E. penicillamine

FILL IN THE BLANK: DRUG NAMES

1. What is a **brand name** for dexamethasone? _____

2. What is the **generic name** for Cortef? _____

3. What is a **brand name** for celecoxib? _____

4. What is the **generic name** for Medrol? _____

5. What is the **brand name** for chloroquine? _____

6. What is the **generic name** for Deltasone (United States) and Winpred (Canada)? _____

7. What is the **brand name** for hydroxychloroquine? _____

8. What is the **generic name** for Imuran? _____

9. What is the **brand name** for mitoxantrone? _____

10. What is a **generic name** for Avonex and Rebif ? _____

11. What is the **generic name** for Cytoxan? _____

12. What is a **brand name** for etanercept? _____

13. What is the **generic name** for Sandimmune and Neoral? _____

14. What is the **brand name** for interferon-beta-1b? _____

15. What is a **brand name** for adalimumab? _____

16. What is the **brand name** for infliximab? _____

17. What is the **brand name** for anakinra? _____

18. What is the **brand name** for leflunomide? _____

Chapter **15 Treatment of Autoimmune Diseases That Affect the Musculoskeletal System**

19. What is a **brand name** for auranofin? _____

20. What is the **generic name** for Cuprimine and Depen? _____

MATCHING

Patient education is an essential component of therapeutics. Select the **best** warning label to apply to the prescription vial given to patients taking the drugs listed.

1. _____ cyclosporine oral solution   A. TAKE ON AN EMPTY STOMACH

2. _____ mitoxantrone   B. AVOID GRAPEFRUIT JUICE

3. _____ methylprednisolone   C. TAKE WITH FOOD

4. _____ hydroxychloroquine   D. AVOID PROLONGED EXPOSURE TO SUNLIGHT

5. _____ penicillamine   E. MAY DISCOLOR URINE

                                               F. TAKE WITH A FULL GLASS OF WATER

TRUE OR FALSE

1. _____ Dermatomyositis affects the muscles of the trunk.

2. _____ Polymyositis is a form of myositis that affects multiple muscles, particularly the muscles closest to the trunk.

3. _____ The reconstituted solution of azathioprine must be shaken well.

4. _____ Cyclosporine oral solution should be dispensed in a glass container.

5. _____ The pharmacy should try to dispense the same manufacturer's product of cyclosporine each time the prescription is refilled.

6. _____ The ending -*mycin* is commonly used for tumor necrosis factor-alpha- inhibitors.

7. _____ Rheumatoid arthritis is far more common in men than in women.

8. _____ Celecoxib is the only selective COX-2 inhibitor still available for use in the United States and Canada.

CRITICAL THINKING

The following hard copies are brought to your pharmacy for filling. Identify the prescription error(s). (You already have the patient's full address on file.)

```
┌─────────────────────────────────────────────┐
│        Kathy Principi, MD      Date _____  │
│           1145 Broadway                        │
│           Anytown, USA                         │
│                                                │
│  Pt. Name _____ Barry Wilcox _____   │
│  Address _____ │
│  ℞  Celebrex 200mg tablets  #30                │
│        i tab daily                             │
│                                                │
│                                                │
│  Refills _____                                │
│     Principi                                   │
│  _____      _____          │
│  Substitution permitted   Dispense as written  │
└─────────────────────────────────────────────┘
```

1. Spot the error in the following

   prescription: _____
   A. Quantity missing
   B. Strength missing
   C. Strength incorrect
   D. Directions incorrect
   E. Dosage form incorrect

```
Kathy Principi, MD        Date _____
        1145 Broadway
        Anytown, USA

Pt. Name _____ Paulette Wilber _____
Address _____

℞   interferon β-1a    #4 prefilled syringes
     inject 0.2ml SC every other day



Refills _____
_____ Principi _____        _____
Substitution permitted         Dispense as written
```

2. Spot the error in the following

   prescription: _____

   A. Quantity missing

   B. Directions incorrect

   C. Strength missing

   D. Strength incorrect

   E. Dosage form incorrect

3. List six pairs of drug names that have look-alike or sound-alike issues with drugs used to treat muscle spasms.

DRUG NAME	LOOK-ALIKE OR SOUND-ALIKE DRUG

RESEARCH ACTIVITY

1. Antibody testing provides an early screening test for some autoimmune diseases. Check the National Library of Medicine website (nlm.nih.gov/medlineplus/rheumatoidarthritis.html#cat1) and other Internet sites, and then write a paragraph explaining the benefit of early diagnosis.

_____

_____

_____

_____

_____

16 Treatment of Osteoporosis and Paget's Disease of the Bone

TERMS AND DEFINITIONS

Match each term with the correct definition below. Some terms may not be used.

A. Bone mineral density

B. Osteoblasts

C. Osteoclasts

D. Osteolysis

E. Osteoporosis

F. Osteopenia

G. Remodeling

H. Bone resorption

1. _____ is a chronic, progressive disease of bone characterized by loss of bone density and increased risk for fractures.

2. The _____ test measures the degree of bone loss.

3. The term used to describe the dissolution or degradation of bone is _____.

4. The term used to describe the process of continual turnover of bone is _____.

5. Decreased bone mineral density, _____, is a precursor of osteoporosis.

6. The process by which bone is broken down to mineral ions (calcium) is called _____.

7. _____ are cells responsible for bone formation, deposition, and mineralization of the collagen matrix of bone.

8. The cells responsible for bone resorption are called _____.

MULTIPLE CHOICE

1. The lifetime risk for fractures in women over 50 years of age is _____.
   A. 1 in 2
   B. 1 in 4
   C. 1 in 10
   D. 1 in 100

2. In a person with osteoporosis, a fragility fracture may occur when the person _____.
   A. falls
   B. coughs
   C. sneezes
   D. is in a car accident
   E. B and C

3. A drug that may cause osteoporosis is

   _____.
   A. Celexa
   B. Celebrex
   C. buspirone
   D. prednisone

4. The percentage of total body calcium located in the

   skeleton is _____.
   A. 10%
   B. 50%
   C. 75%
   D. 99%
   E. 100%

5. Which hormone is *not* involved in the regulation of

   serum calcium levels? _____
   A. Parathyroid hormone
   B. Glucagon
   C. Calcitonin
   D. Vitamin D

6. A program for the prevention and treatment of
   osteoporosis includes all of the following *except*

   _____.
   A. vitamin A
   B. consumption of foods rich in calcium
   C. vitamin D
   D. weight-bearing exercise
   E. pharmacotherapy

7. Which drug must be taken on an empty stomach at
   least 30 minutes before the first meal or beverage of

   the day? _____
   A. calcium
   B. Evista
   C. Fosamax
   D. Estrace

8. Patients taking Didronel and Aredia must sit upright

   or stand for at least _____ minutes
   after dosing to avoid possible esophageal ulceration.
   A. 30
   B. 60
   C. 90
   D. 120

9. Select the calcium supplement that contains the
   highest percentage of elemental calcium per tablet.

   _____
   A. calcium chloride
   B. calcium citrate
   C. calcium lactate
   D. calcium carbonate
   E. calcium gluconate

10. The use of teriparatide, a genetically engineered
    form of human parathyroid hormone and the only
    drug currently available in this category, is limited

    because of risks for _____.
    A. fractures
    B. osteosarcoma
    C. pituitary tumors
    D. all of the above

FILL IN THE BLANK: DRUG NAMES

1. What is a *brand name* for pamidronate? _____

2. What is the *generic name* for Actonel? _____

3. What is a *brand name* for alendronate? _____

4. What is the *generic name* for Skelid (United States)? _____

5. What is the *brand name* for etidronate? _____

6. What is the *generic name* for Zometa? _____

7. What is the *brand name* for raloxifene? _____

8. What is the *generic name* for Fosamax Plus D (United States)? _____

9. What is a *generic name* for Actonel with Calcium (United States)? _____

10. What is the *generic name* for Miacalcin nasal spray? _____

11. What is a *generic name* for CombiPatch (United States) and Estalis (Canada)? _____

12. What is the *generic name* for Climara? _____

13. What is the *brand name* for conjugated estrogens? _____

14. What is the *generic name* for Premphase and Prempro? _____

15. What a *brand name* for estrogens esterified? _____

16. What is the *generic name* for Ogen? _____

17. What is the *generic name* for Forteo (United States? _____

MATCHING

Patient education is an essential component of therapeutics. Select the **best** warning label to apply to the prescription vial given to patients taking the drugs listed.

1. _____ Actonel   A. ROTATE SITE OF APPLICATION

2. _____ Climara   B. STORE IN MANUFACTURER'S SEALED FOIL POUCH

3. _____ Premarin   C. TAKE WITH FOOD

4. _____ CombiPatch   D. TAKE 30 MINUTES BEFORE THE FIRST MEAL OF THE DAY

MATCHING

Match each drug to its pharmacological classification.

1. _____ Premarin   A. bisphosphonate

2. _____ Evista   B. selective estrogen receptor modulator

3. _____ Forteo   C. estrogen replacement

4. _____ Fosamax   D. anabolic agent

TRUE OR FALSE

1. _____ The rate of bone loss for men and women is equal after age 65 to 70 years.

2. _____ Hormones linked to the regulation of bone formation and bone loss are estrogen, progesterone, and luteinizing hormone.

3. _____ Paget's disease is characterized by insufficient bone resorption.

4. _____ Paget's disease is most common in women older than 55 years.

5. _____ Secondary osteoporosis may be caused by diseases or drugs.

The following hard copies are brought to your pharmacy for filling. Identify the prescription error(s). (You already have the patient's full address on file.)

Kathy Principi, MD   Date _____
1145 Broadway
Anytown, USA

Pt. Name _____ Belinda Wilcox _____

Address _____

℞   *Miacalcin nasal spray   1 bottle*
       1 spray in each nostril daily

Refills _____

____ *Principi* ____   _____

Substitution permitted   Dispense as written

---

1. Spot the error in the following prescription:

   _____

   A. Quantity missing
   B. Strength missing
   C. Strength incorrect
   D. Directions incorrect
   E. Dosage form incorrect

Kathy Principi, MD   Date _____
1145 Broadway
Anytown, USA

Pt. Name _____ Paulette Wilber _____

Address _____

℞   *Fosamax 70mg once weekly*

Refills _____

____ *Principi* ____   _____

Substitution permitted   Dispense as written

---

2. Spot the error in the following prescription:

   _____

   A. Quantity missing
   B. Directions incorrect
   C. Strength missing
   D. Strength incorrect
   E. Dosage form incorrect

---

3. List six pairs of drug names that have look-alike or sound-alike issues with drugs used to treat muscle spasms.

DRUG NAME	LOOK-ALIKE OR SOUND-ALIKE DRUG

1. Access the National Library of Medicine website (nlm.nih.gov/medlineplus/osteoporosis.html) and other Internet sites, and then write a paragraph justifying the following recommendation: "It is best to lay the foundation for healthy dense bones early in life."

_____

_____

_____

_____

_____

17 Treatment of Hyperuricemia and Gout

TERMS AND DEFINITIONS

Match each term with the correct definition below. Some terms may not be used.

A. Gout

B. Hyperuricemia

C. Urates

D. Uricosuric

E. Purine

1. A product of purine metabolism that produces inflammation is _____.

2. A drug that increases the renal clearance of urates is _____.

3. _____ is a disease associated with deposits of urate crystals in the joints.

4. _____ is a condition in which urate levels build up in the blood serum.

5. _____ is one of two nitrogen-containing bases found in DNA and RNA.

MULTIPLE CHOICE

1. Hyperuricemia is associated with all of the following conditions *except* _____.
   A. hypertension
   B. kidney disease
   C. hyperlipidemia
   D. osteoporosis
   E. obesity and insulin resistance

2. Deposits of uric acid are called _____.
   A. tophi
   B. cysts
   C. keloids
   D. tumors

3. Gout is most common in _____.
   A. children
   B. men
   C. women
   D. adolescents

4. Acute gout attacks will resolve spontaneously in _____ days without treatment.
   A. 1 to 2
   B. 3 to 6
   C. 7 to 10
   D. 10 to 14

5. Which joint(s) is (are) *not* commonly affected by gout? _____
   A. Big toe, foot, and ankle
   B. Knee
   C. Neck
   D. Wrist and finger
   E. Elbow

6. Which drug would *not* be prescribed for the treatment of gout? _____
   A. colchicine
   B. probenecid
   C. allopurinol
   D. hydrochlorothiazide
   E. indomethacin

7. Which drug blocks the final enzymatic step in the production of uric acid? _____
   A. colchicine
   B. probenecid
   C. allopurinol
   D. hydrochlorothiazide
   E. celecoxib

8. Which foods and beverages may increase the likelihood of a gout attack? _____
   A. Beer and fish
   B. Milk and cheese
   C. Pasta and tomato sauce
   D. Rice and potatoes

9. A common side effect of colchicine is _____.
   A. tremors
   B. nausea and vomiting
   C. ataxia
   D. constipation

10. Drugs prescribed for the treatment of gout include _____.
    A. analgesics
    B. anti-inflammatories
    C. uricosurics and inhibitors of uric acid synthesis
    D. A, B, and C

FILL IN THE BLANK: DRUG NAMES

1. What is a **brand name** for colchicine? _____

2. What is the **generic name** for Orudis? _____

3. What is a **brand name** for methylprednisolone? _____

4. What is the **generic name** for Benuryl? _____

5. What is the **brand name** for allopurinol? _____

6. What is the **generic name** for Krystexxa? _____

7. What is the **brand name** for febuxostat? _____

MATCHING

Patient education is an essential component of therapeutics. Select the **best** warning label to apply to the prescription vial given to patients taking the drugs listed.

1. _____ Zyloprim 300 mg   A. AVOID ALCOHOL

2. _____ colchicine 0.6 mg   B. AVOID ASPIRIN

3. _____ probenecid 500 mg   C. MAY CAUSE DIZZINESS OR DROWSINESS

MATCHING

Match each drug to its pharmacological classification.

1. _____ Zyloprim   A. Anti-inflammatory

2. _____ colchicine   B. Uricosuric

3. _____ probenecid   C. Inhibitor of uric acid synthesis

TRUE OR FALSE

1. _____ Shellfish and bacon are high in purines.

2. _____ The brand name of allopurinol is Zyrtec.

3. _____ Probenecid and allopurinol should be taken on an empty stomach.

4. _____ A uricosuric is a drug that decreases the renal clearance of urates.

5. _____ The principal anti-inflammatory used in the treatment of gout is colchicine.

CRITICAL THINKING

The following hard copies are brought to your pharmacy for filling. Identify the prescription error(s). (You already have the patient's full address on file.)

```
        Kathy Principi, MD      Date _____
          1145 Broadway
          Seattle, WA 98122
Pt. Name _____ Belinda Wilcox _____
Address _____

Rx   Colchine 6.0mg    #30
     1-2 tabs every 1-2 hours until relief or 3 doses.



Refills _____

_____ Principi _____          _____
Substitution permitted        Dispense as written
```

1. Spot the error in the following prescription:

   _____

   A. Quantity missing
   B. Strength missing
   C. Strength incorrect
   D. Directions incorrect
   E. Dosage form incorrect

```
        Kathy Principi, MD      Date _____
          1145 Broadway
          Seattle, WA 98122
Pt. Name _____ Paulette Wilber _____
Address _____

Rx   Zyloprim 100mg
     Start with 100mg/day and increase to 200mg/day



Refills _____

_____ Principi _____          _____
Substitution permitted        Dispense as written
```

2. Spot the error in the following prescription:

   _____

   A. Quantity missing
   B. Directions incorrect
   C. Strength missing
   D. Strength incorrect
   E. Dosage form incorrect

3. List six pairs of drug names that have look-alike or sound-alike issues with drugs used to treat gout or hyperuricemia.

DRUG NAME	LOOK-ALIKE OR SOUND-ALIKE DRUG

RESEARCH ACTIVITY

1. Persons with gout will be advised to make lifestyle changes to reduce their risk for gout attacks. Check the National Library of Medicine website and other Internet sites to do research on gout and hyperuricemia (nlm.nih .gov/medlineplus/gout.html). Write a paragraph explaining what people with gout can do to stay healthy and avoid gout attacks.

_____

_____

_____

_____

_____

18 Treatment of Glaucoma

TERMS AND DEFINITIONS

Match each term with the correct definition below. Some terms may not be used.

A. Aqueous humor

B. Central vision

C. Cornea

D. Conjunctiva

E. Angle-closure glaucoma

F. Open-angle glaucoma

G. Intraocular pressure

H. Keratotomy

I. Lacrimal apparatus

J. Optic disk

K. Optic nerve

L. Peripheral vision

M. Tonometry

N. Trabecular meshwork

O. Iris

1. _____ is a disorder characterized by elevated pressure in the eye; it can lead to permanent blindness.

2. The region of the _____ where the retinal nerve fibers from the eye exit and the blood vessels enter the eye is called the _____.

3. _____ are structures that keep the surface of the eye moistened with tears.

4. The _____ is the clear part of the eye located in front of the iris.

5. The fluid that is made in the front part of the eye is called _____.

6. _____ is what is seen when you look straight ahead or when you read.

7. Schlemm's canal, or the _____, is made up of small openings around the outer edge of the iris that form meshlike drainage canals.

8. _____ is sometimes called "side vision."

9. The term for a procedure in which an incision is made in the cornea to correct myopia is _____.

10. _____ is an examination that uses a device to measure the pressure in the eye.

11. The _____ is a transparent mucous membrane that lines each lid and continues over the surface of the eyeball.

12. _____ is characterized by a sudden increase in intraocular pressure caused by obstruction of the drainage portal between the cornea and the iris (angle).

13. _____ is the colored part of the eye that can expand or contract to allow the right amount of light to enter the eye.

MULTIPLE CHOICE

1. _____ is usually the first area of vision to be lost with glaucoma.
   A. Peripheral vision
   B. Near vision
   C. Far vision
   D. Central vision

2. Carbonic anhydrase inhibitors may cause allergic reactions in people that have allergies to
   _____ anti-infective agents.
   A. penicillin
   B. tetracycline
   C. sulfonamide
   D. macrolide

3. A common ending for prostaglandin analogues is
   _____.
   A. -prost
   B. -zolamide
   C. =triptyline
   D. -pramine

4. The mechanism of action for drugs used in the treatment of glaucoma is _____.
   A. to increase the formation of aqueous humor
   B. to decrease the formation of aqueous humor
   C. to promote the drainage of aqueous humor
   D. to decrease the drainage of aqueous humor
   E. B and C

5. All of the following drug classifications decrease formation of the aqueous humor *except*
   _____.
   A. beta blockers
   B. prostaglandin analogues
   C. alpha-adrenergic agonists
   D. carbonic anhydrase inhibitors

6. Which carbonic anhydrase inhibitor is administered orally? _____
   A. acetazolamide
   B. brinzolamide
   C. Trusopt
   D. Cosopt

7. Most ophthalmic drugs used for the treatment of glaucoma require contact lens wearers to wait at least
   _____ before reinserting their contact lenses.
   A. 5 minutes
   B. 10 minutes
   C. 15 minutes
   D. 30 minutes

8. Which glaucoma eye drops must be stored in the refrigerator? _____
   A. Xalatan
   B. Lumigan
   C. Pilopine HS gel
   D. Propine

FILL IN THE BLANK: DRUG NAMES

1. What is a **brand name** for betaxolol? _____

2. What is the **generic name** for Betagan? _____

3. What is a **brand name** for timolol maleate? _____

4. What is the **generic name** for Iopidine? _____

5. What is the **generic name** for Diamox? _____

6. What is the **brand name** for timolol plus latanoprost? _____

7. What is the **generic name** for Azopt? _____

8. What is the **generic name** for Alphagan? _____

9. What is the **generic name** for Trusopt? _____

10. What is the **brand name** for travoprost? _____

11. What is the **brand name** for dorzolamide and timolol? _____

12. What is the **generic name** for Isopto Carbachol? _____

13. What is the **brand name** for bimatoprost? _____

14. What is the **generic name** for Pilopine? _____

15. What is the **brand name** for latanoprost? _____

16. What is the **generic name** for Phospholine Iodide (United States)? _____

MATCHING

Match each drug to its pharmacological classification.

1. _____ Timoptic   A. Alpha-adrenergic agonist

2. _____ Alphagan   B. Cholinergic agonist

3. _____ dorzolamide   C. Prostaglandin analogue

4. _____ latanoprost   D. Carbonic anhydrase inhibitor

5. _____ Pilocar   E. Beta-adrenergic antagonist

TRUE OR FALSE

1. _____ The iris is the colored part of the eye that contracts to allow the right amount of light to enter the eye.

2. _____ The ending *-zolamide* is commonly used for carbonic anhydrase inhibitors.

3. _____ Pharmacy technicians are susceptible to "dry eyes" while performing sterile preparation of intravenous products in a laminar flow hood.

4. _____ Glaucoma is the leading cause of blindness worldwide.

5. _____ The risk for glaucoma decreases with age.

6. _____ Open-angle glaucoma is more common than angle-closure glaucoma.

7. _____ Miotics are drugs that dilate the pupil.

CRITICAL THINKING

The following hard copies are brought to your pharmacy for filling. Identify the prescription error(s). (You already have the patient's full address on file.)

```
┌─────────────────────────────────────────┐
│      Kathy Principi, MD      Date _____ │
│         1145 Broadway                    │
│         Anytown, USA                     │
│                                          │
│ Pt. Name _____ Ellen Wilcox _____  │
│ Address _____  │
│ ℞   Xalatan 0.005%   2.5ml               │
│     Instill one drop                     │
│                                          │
│                                          │
│ Refills _____                           │
│ ____ Principi ____    _____  │
│ Substitution permitted   Dispense as written │
└─────────────────────────────────────────┘
```

1. Spot the error in the following prescription:

   _____

   A. Quantity missing
   B. Directions incomplete
   C. Strength missing
   D. Strength incorrect
   E. Dosage form incorrect

2. List three pairs of drug names that have look-alike or sound-alike issues with drugs used to treat glaucoma.

DRUG NAME	LOOK-ALIKE OR SOUND-ALIKE DRUG

RESEARCH ACTIVITY

1. According to World Health Organization (WHO) data, glaucoma is one of the leading causes of blindness globally, and the prevalence is rising. Check the WHO website (who.int/blindness/causes/priority/en/index7.html) to do research on glaucoma to try to explain why. Can this trend be reversed?

_____

_____

_____

_____

_____

19 Treatment of Disorders of the Ear

TERMS AND DEFINITIONS

Match each term with the correct definition below. Some terms may not be used.

A. Cerumen

B. Cochlea

C. Conductive hearing loss

D. Equilibrium

E. Labyrinth

F. Ménière's disease

G. Otitis media

H. Otosclerosis

I. Ototoxicity

J. Presbycusis

K. Saccule

L. Tinnitus

M. Utricle

N. Vertigo

O. Otitis

P. Otoliths

Q. Tympanic membrane

1. Bilateral hearing loss, or _____, is linked to aging and often accompanied by tinnitus.

2. _____ is an inflammation of the middle ear.

3. The waxlike substance secreted by modified sweat glands in the ear is called _____.

4. _____, the feeling of spinning in space, is a symptom of _____, a chronic inner ear disease associated with intermittent buildup of fluid in the inner ear.

5. The _____ is a portion of the inner ear involved in hearing.

6. A term that describes damage or toxicity to the ear or eighth cranial nerve is _____.

7. Abnormalities of the outer ear or middle ear that interfere with transmission of sound between the inner ear and outer ear may cause _____.

8. The _____, a bony structure in the inner ear, is involved in maintaining _____, or balance.

9. Symptoms of _____ are intermittent or continuous whistling, crackling, squeaking, or ringing in the ears.

10. The term that describes the hardening of the bones of the middle ear is _____.

11. The structures in the inner ear responsible for sensing motion are the labyrinth, _____, and _____.

12. _____ is inflammation of the ear.

13. _____ is known as the eardrum.

14. _____ is calcium carbonate crystals found in the utricle and saccule of the inner ear.

MULTIPLE CHOICE

1. Select the **false** statement. _____
   A. Otosclerosis is an autoimmune disease.
   B. Otosclerosis may cause hearing loss and tinnitus.
   C. Otosclerosis is a disorder that causes destruction of bone in the ear.
   D. Otosclerosis is also called Ménière's disease.

2. Drugs that may cause tinnitus are _____.
   A. aspirin and alcohol
   B. diphenhydramine and scopolamine
   C. diazepam and triazolam
   D. metocarbamol and cyclobenzaprine

3. Which of the following conditions is *not* linked to vertigo? _____
   A. Ménière's disease
   B. Benign paroxysmal positional vertigo
   C. Gout
   D. Head trauma
   E. Infection

4. Symptoms of vertigo include all of the following *except* _____.
   A. dizziness
   B. nausea
   C. muscle weakness
   D. blurred vision
   E. disorientation

5. Meclizine should be used with caution in _____.
   A. patients with prostate disease
   B. patients with asthma
   C. lactating women
   D. A, B, and C

6. Which is *not* a property of cerumen?
   _____
   A. Antiviral
   B. Bactericidal
   C. Water repellant
   D. Lubricant

7. Carbamide peroxide 6.5% is the only approved agent for _____ removal.
   A. cerumen (ear wax)
   B. water or fluid
   C. bacteria
   D. foreign material

8. Which product is used to treat swimmer's ear?
   _____
   A. meclizine
   B. carbamide peroxide
   C. isopropyl alcohol 95% and glycerin 5%
   D. scopolamine hydrobromide

FILL IN THE BLANK: DRUG NAMES

1. What is the *generic name* for Serc (Canada)? _____

2. What is the *generic name* for Antivert? _____

3. What is the *generic name* for Transderm Scop (United States) and Transderm V (Canada)?

   _____

4. What is the *generic name* for Auralgan? _____

5. What is the *generic name* for Auro-Dri Ear Drying Aid? _____

6. What is the *generic name* for Debrox and Murine Ear Wax Removal System? _____

TRUE OR FALSE

1. _____ Otitis externa is an infection of the middle ear.

2. _____ The tympanic membrane is commonly known as the eardrum.

3. _____ Otoliths are calcium carbonate crystals found in the inner ear.

4. _____ A commonly used ending for local anesthetics is *-caine*.

5. _____ Our perception of balance and movement is a function of input from the eye, inner ear, and sense receptors on the skin and skeleton.

6. _____ When the ear is inflamed, otic suspensions are more soothing than solutions that contain alcohol.

CRITICAL THINKING

The following hard copies are brought to your pharmacy for filling. Identify the prescription error(s). (You already have the patient's full address on file.)

```
Kathy Principi, MD          Date _____
1145 Broadway
Anytown, USA

Pt. Name _____ Ellen Wilber _____
Address _____
R̆   Antivert 25mg      1 bottle
     2 tablets BID



Refills _____
_____Principi_____        _____
Substitution permitted    Dispense as written
```

1. Spot the error in the following prescription:

   _____

   A. Quantity missing
   B. Directions incomplete
   C. Strength missing
   D. Strength incorrect
   E. Dosage form incorrect

2. List one pair of drug names that have look-alike or sound-alike issues with drugs used to treat vertigo.

DRUG NAME	LOOK-ALIKE OR SOUND-ALIKE DRUG

RESEARCH ACTIVITY

1. Treatment of balance disorders may involve physical therapy, diet, and lifestyle changes. What diet and lifestyle changes might be recommended?

_____

_____

_____

_____

_____

20 Treatment of Ophthalmic and Otic Infections

TERMS AND DEFINITIONS

Match each term with the correct definition below. Some terms may not be used.

A. Blepharitis

B. Conjunctivitis (pink eye)

C. Cytomegalovirus retinitis

D. Vitreous floaters

E. Helminthes

F. Fusarium keratitis

G. Otorrhea

H. Photopsia

I. Stye

J. Uveitis

K. Herpes zoster ophthalmicus

L. Otitis media

M. Otitis externa

N. Keratitis

O. Iritis

P. Herpes simplex keratitis

1. Particles that appear as spots, cobwebs, or spiders in the retina are called _____.

2. _____ is a viral opportunistic infection of the eye.

3. The term used to describe a discharge coming from the external auditory canal or inside of the canal is
_____.

4. _____ is a severe infection of the cornea that may be caused by bacteria or fungi.

5. A serious eye condition, _____ produces inflammation of the uvea.

6. _____ is a condition similar to floaters and associated with flashes of light.

7. _____ is a chronic disease that is characterized by flaky scales that form on the eyelids and eyelashes.

8. A(n) _____ is an acute self-limiting infection that causes a painful lump to form on the eyelid margin.

9. The common, self-limiting ailment known as _____ is commonly called pink eye.

10. _____ are parasitic worms.

11. _____ is a condition associated with inflammation of the iris.

12. _____ is a painful eye infection caused by the herpesvirus that can lead to blindness.

13. _____ is a rare fungal infection that occurs in soft contact lens wearers and can result in blindness.

14. _____ is the inflammation of the ear canal or external ear.

15. _____ is the inflammation of the middle ear typically caused by a viral or bacterial infection.

MULTIPLE CHOICE

1. _____ is a rare fungal infection that occurs in soft contact lens wearers and can result in blindness.
   A. Fusarium keratitis
   B. Cytomegalovirus keratitis
   C. Herpes simplex keratitis
   D. Herpes zoster keratitis

2. Which eye infection does *not* lead to blindness if untreated? _____
   A. Uveitis
   B. Stye
   C. Keratitis
   D. Onchocerciasis

3. Uveitis is treated with the administration of
   _____.
   A. corticosteroids (to reduce inflammation)
   B. mydriatics (to reduce painful swelling)
   C. anti-infectives or antivirals as appropriate
   D. A, B, and C

4. Blepharitis is treated by applying clean warm compresses to the eyelids and applying
   _____.
   A. Tobrex ointment
   B. boric acid ointment
   C. Viroptic
   D. Timoptic

5. Which drug is *not* administered to treat cytomegalovirus retinitis? _____
   A. ganciclovir
   B. dipivefrin
   C. valganciclovir
   D. foscarnet
   E. cidofovir

6. Select the **false** statement. _____
   A. Ocular toxoplasmosis is caused by viral infection.
   B. Toxoplasmosis is transmitted by handling or eating raw or undercooked meat.
   C. Toxoplasmosis can be transmitted by handling cat feces.
   D. Toxoplasmosis is treated by administering pyrimethamine and sulfonamides (e.g., sulfadiazine).

7. Which drug is used to treat toxocariasis?
   _____
   A. sulfamethoxazole plus trimethoprim
   B. thiobendazole
   C. ganciclovir
   D. valganciclovir

8. Which self-care activity may produce otitis externa?
   _____
   A. Drying ears well after swimming
   B. Digging ear wax out of the ear with cotton swabs
   C. Avoiding areas with excessive moisture or heat
   D. A and C

FILL IN THE BLANK: DRUG NAMES

1. What is a *brand name* for tobramycin? _____

2. What is the *generic name* for Garamycin (Canada) and Gentopic (United States)? _____

3. What is the *brand name* for sulfacetamide Na$^+$? _____

4. What is the *generic name* for Polytrim? _____

5. What is the *generic name* for Ciloxan? _____

6. What is the *generic name* for Ocuflox and Floxin Otic? _____

7. What is the *generic name* for Iquix (United States)? _____

8. What is the *brand name* for sulfacetamide plus prednisolone acetate? _____

9. What is the *generic name* for Maxitrol? _____

10. What is the *brand name* for tobramycin plus dexamethasone? _____

11. What is the *generic name* for Poly-Pred (United States)? _____

12. What is the *brand name* for ganciclovir? _____

13. What is the *generic name* for Viroptic? _____

14. What is the *brand name* for valganciclovir? _____

15. What is the *generic name* for Natacyn (United States)? _____

16. What is the *brand name* for albendazole? _____

17. What is the *generic name* for Cortisporin? _____

MATCHING

Match each drug to its use.

1. _____ albendazole

2. _____ Viroptic

3. _____ natamycin

4. _____ Tobradex

A. Parasitic eye infections

B. Bacterial eye infections

C. Viral eye infections

D. Fungal eye infections

TRUE OR FALSE

1. _____ Iritis is a condition associated with inflammation of the cornea.

2. _____ Onchocerciasis is also known as river blindness.

3. _____ Helminthes are fungi that can cause eye infection and blindness.

4. _____ Pink eye causes itching, burning, and teary outflow.

5. _____ Conjunctivitis (pink eye) may be caused by a virus or bacteria.

6. _____ Bacterial resistance is reduced by regular use of anti-infective agents to treat otitis media.

7. _____ Cortisporin is marketed as an otic solution and ophthalmic solution.

CRITICAL THINKING

The following hard copies are brought to your pharmacy for filling. Identify the prescription error(s). (You already have the patient's full address on file.)

| Kathy Principi, MD Date _____ |
| 1145 Broadway |
| Anytown, USA |
| |
| Pt. Name _____ Elisa Weinberg _____ |
| Address _____ |
| ℞ *Tobrex 0.3%*   *5ml* |
| *apply ointment 2-3 times a day* |
| |
| Refills _____ |
| _____ *Principi* _____ |
| Substitution permitted   Dispense as written |

1. Spot the error in the following prescription:

   _____

   A. Quantity missing
   B. Directions incomplete
   C. Strength missing
   D. Strength incorrect
   E. Dosage form incorrect

2. List three pairs of drug names that have look-alike or sound-alike issues with drugs used to treat ophthalmic and otic infections.

DRUG NAME	LOOK-ALIKE OR SOUND-ALIKE DRUG

RESEARCH ACTIVITY

1. Anti-infective agents have routinely been administered to treat acute infections of otitis media and then continued prophylactically. Recently, this policy has been questioned. Check the National Library of Medicine website (nlm.nih.gov/medlineplus/earinfections.html) and other websites and do research on the treatment of ear infections. Write a paragraph explaining why the trend may be shifting away from routine use of anti-infectives.

_____

_____

_____

_____

_____

21 | Treatment of Angina

TERMS AND DEFINITIONS

Match each term with the correct definition below. Some terms may not be used.

A. Angina pectoris

B. Arteriosclerosis

C. Atheroma

D. Atherosclerosis

E. Coronary artery disease

F. Hyperlipidemia

G. Ischemia

H. Ischemic heart disease

I. Necrosis

J. Plaque

K. Thrombus

L. Vasospasms

M. Embolus

N. Myocardial infarction

O. Arterial plaque

1. _____ is a condition that occurs when the arteries that supply blood to the heart muscle become hardened and narrowed.

2. Myocardial _____ is a deficient blood supply to the heart.

3. A(n) _____ is a hardened lipid streak or _____ that has formed within an artery.

4. An ischemic heart disease, _____ is characterized by a severe squeezing or pressure-like thoracic pain brought on by exertion or stress.

5. _____ is the term used to describe cell death and may be caused by lack of blood and oxygen to an affected area.

6. _____ is a condition where there is an increased concentration of cholesterol and triglycerides in the blood.

7. A stationary blood clot is called a _____.

8. _____ is any condition in which heart muscle is damaged or works inefficiently because of an absence or relative deficiency of its blood supply.

9. _____ is a process in which plaques containing cholesterol, lipid material, and lipophages are formed within arteries.

10. Symptoms of angina may be caused by _____ that constrict blood vessels and reduce the flow of blood and oxygen.

11. _____ is a condition where artery walls thicken and lose their elasticity.

12. _____ is a hardened lipid streak within an artery formed by deposits of cholesterol, lipid material, and lipophages.

13. A(n) _____ is a moving clot.

14. _____ is also referred to as a "heart attack"; it results in heart muscle tissue death and is caused by the occlusion of a coronary artery.

MULTIPLE CHOICE

1. Risk factors for angina include all of the following except _____.
   A. smoking
   B. a diet high in cholesterol and salt
   C. excessive alcohol consumption
   D. mild exercise
   E. obesity

2. All of the following drugs are used in the treatment of angina except _____.
   A. nitrates
   B. diuretics
   C. beta-blocking drugs
   D. Ca^2 channel blockers

3. A woman was awakened in the middle of the night with severe chest pain. Her physician prescribed sublingual nitroglycerin. Which of the following adverse reactions is associated with sublingual nitroglycerin? _____
   A. Flushing of the skin
   B. Headache
   C. Stinging under the tongue
   D. A, B, and C

4. A common ending for beta-adrenergic blockers is _____.
   A. -dipine
   B. -olol
   C. -mycin
   D. -zosin

5. Patients using nitroglycerin transdermal patches should be advised to _____.
   A. wear the patch for 24 hours each day
   B. apply a patch at the onset of symptoms of angina
   C. rotate the sites on the skin to prevent skin irritation
   D. apply the patch directly over the heart

6. Which drug may be taken concurrently with nitroglycerin? _____
   A. Viagra
   B. Cialis
   C. Tenormin
   D. Levitra

7. Isosorbide mononitrate is _____.
    A. manufactured in a transdermal patch dosage form
    B. used to treat acute symptoms of angina
    C. used to prevent symptoms of angina
    D. manufactured as a sublingual tablet

8. Which statement about beta-adrenergic blockers is

    false? _____
    A. Beta-adrenergic blockers reduce the heart's demand for oxygen.
    B. Beta-adrenergic blockers decrease the frequency and severity of stable angina.
    C. Beta-adrenergic blockers increase the heart's demand for oxygen.
    D. Beta-adrenergic blockers are contraindicated in patients with asthma and diabetes.

9. Which drug is effective in reducing vasospasms

    associated with variant angina? _____
    A. propranolol
    B. atenolol
    C. nitroglycerin
    D. nifedipine

FILL IN THE BLANK: DRUG NAMES

1. What is a *brand name* for isosorbide mononitrate? _____

2. What is the *generic name* for Dilatrate-SR (United States) and Cedocard-SR (Canada)?

    _____

3. What is a *brand name* for nitroglycerin patches? _____

4. What is a *brand name* for nitroglycerin SL? _____

5. What is the *brand name* for atenolol? _____

6. What is the *generic name* for Lopressor? _____

7. What is a *brand name* for propranolol? _____

8. What is the *generic name* for Corgard (United States)? _____

9. What is the *brand name* for amlodipine? _____

10. What is the *generic name* for Cardizem and Tiazac? _____

11. What is the *generic name* for Procardia (United States) and Adalat? _____

12. What is the *generic name* for Cardene (United States)? _____

13. What is the *generic name* for Covera and Isoptin? _____

MATCHING

Patient education is an essential component of therapeutics. Select the best warning label to apply to the prescription vial given to patients taking the drugs listed.

1. _____ Isordil 10 mg

2. _____ Minitran

3. _____ NitroLingual

4. _____ nitroglycerin 0.4 mg SL

5. _____ Imdur

A. STORE IN ORIGINAL CONTAINER

B. SWALLOW WHOLE; DO NOT CRUSH OR CHEW

C. ROTATE SITE OF APPLICATION

D. HOLD SPRAY IN MOUTH AT LEAST 10 SECONDS BEFORE SWALLOWING

E. TAKE ON AN EMPTY STOMACH

MATCHING

Match the nitroglycerin dosage form with its therapeutic use.

1. _____ nitroglycerin SL

2. _____ nitroglycerin patch

3. _____ nitroglycerin capsule

4. _____ nitroglycerin spray

5. _____ nitroglycerin ointment

A. Used for relief of acute anginal attacks

B. Used for prevention of anginal attacks

MATCHING

Match each drug to its pharmacological classification.

1. _____ Tenormin

2. _____ Imdur

3. _____ verapamil

A. Nitrate

B. Beta blocker

C. Calcium channel blocker

TRUE OR FALSE

1. _____ Atherosclerosis is sometimes called "hardening of the arteries."

2. _____ Nitroglycerin should always be dispensed without a safety cap for easy access.

3. _____ All nitrates have *-nitro* or *-nitra* in their brand or generic name.

4. _____ Cardizem 180 mg is available in XR, XT, CD, and SR dosage forms.

5. _____ Unstable angina may occur at rest.

6. _____ Stable angina may be precipitated by eating heavy meals, exposure to extreme changes in temperature, and emotional stress.

7. _____ Nitroglycerin SL tablets may be dispensed in amber plastic prescription vials.

CRITICAL THINKING

The following hard copies are brought to your pharmacy for filling. Identify the prescription error(s). (You already have the patient's full address on file.)

Marc Cordova, MD   Date _____
1145 Broadway
Anytown, USA

Pt. Name _____ Carlton Peak _____
Address _____

Rx   nitroglycerin 6.5mg cap
     i BID

Refills _____
____ Cordova ____   _____
Substitution permitted   Dispense as written

---

1. Spot the prescription error: _____
   A. Quantity missing
   B. Strength missing
   C. Strength incorrect
   D. Directions incorrect
   E. Dosage form incorrect

Marc Cordova, MD   Date _____
1145 Broadway
Anytown, USA

Pt. Name _____ Bill Chris _____
Address _____

Rx   transdermal NTG   #30
     1 q AM remove in 12 hours

Refills _____
____ Cordova ____   _____
Substitution permitted   Dispense as written

---

2. Spot the prescription error: _____
   A. Quantity missing
   B. Strength missing
   C. Directions missing
   D. Directions incorrect
   E. Dosage form incorrect

Anh Dang Tu, MD   Date _____
1145 Broadway
Anytown, USA

Pt. Name _____ Loan Nguyen _____
Address _____

Rx   isosorbide mononitrite 30mg tab
     i sl prn chest pain   #30

Refills _____
_____   ____ Tu ____
Substitution permitted   Dispense as written

---

3. Spot the prescription error: _____
   A. Quantity missing
   B. Strength missing
   C. Strength incorrect
   D. Directions incorrect
   E. Dosage form incorrect

4. List six pairs of drug names that have look-alike or sound-alike issues with drugs used to treat migraine headache or angina.

DRUG NAME	LOOK-ALIKE OR SOUND-ALIKE DRUG

5. Write a short paragraph describing the relationship between coronary arteries, exertional angina, and vasospastic angina.

_____

_____

_____

_____

_____

RESEARCH ACTIVITY

1. Hector Carvajal calls to renew his antianginal medication. He does not remember the name of the drug. Review his patient profile, and then make a list of the medications that are used in the treatment of angina. Develop a list of questions you might ask to identify the drug he is requesting.

Last name: Carvajal	First name: Hector	Gender: M
Address: 1906 E Denny Wy	City: Anytown	DOB: 4-12-49
Allergies: penicillin	Disc.:	Phone: 222-322-6789
Comment: $8/12 copay		
Insurance: PC	Plan: 05	Group:12345678
ID#: 526458904	Copay: $8.00	
Cardholder: Rivera	Jorge	Exp. date:

DATE	RX#	DRUG AND STRENGTH	SIG	QTY	MD	RF
1-1-08	72345	HCTZ 50 mg	1 QD	100	Johnson, C	2
1-1-08	72346	Slow K 8 mEq	1 BID	60	Johnson, C	3
1-2-08	79278	Nitrostat 0.4 mg	1 sl PRN	60	Johnson, C	1
2-24-08	81956	Cotrim DS	1 BID	20	Principi, K	
2-24-08	84358	Hycotuss	5 mL q6h	120	Principi, K	
3-2-08	72346	Slow K 8 mEq	1 BID	100	Johnson, C	2
3-2-08	79278	Imdur 30 mg	1 QD	60	Johnson, C	1
4-1-08	96346	enalapril 25 mg	1 BID	60	Johnson, C	2
4-7-08	102344	Nitrostat 0.4 mg	1 sl PRN	100	Johnson, C	4
4-10-08	105278	NitroDur 5 cm^2/24 hours	1 QD	30	Johnson, C	1

ANTIANGINAL DRUG	DRUG IDENTIFICATION QUESTIONS
	1.
	2.
	3.

2. Hector claims that NitroDur irritates him. What may be responsible for the irritation?

_____

_____

_____

_____

_____

Treatment of Hypertension

TERMS AND DEFINITIONS

Match each term with the correct definition below. Some terms may not be used.

A. Aldosterone

B. Angiotensin II

C. Angiotensin-converting enzyme (ACE)

D. Cardiac output

E. Diastolic blood pressure (DBP)

F. Diuretic

G. Hyperkalemia

H. Hypokalemia

I. Hypertension (high blood pressure)

J. Orthostatic hypotension

K. Photosensitivity

L. Prehypertension

M. Peripheral vascular resistance

N. Renin–aldosterone–angiotensin system (RAAS)

O. Systolic blood pressure (SBP)

P. Body mass index

Q. Gynecomastia

R. Hirsutism

S. Hypernatremia

T. Hyponatremia

U. Hyperuricemia

V. Isolated systolic hypertension

W. Metabolic syndrome

X. Nocturia

Y. Preeclampsia

1. A potent vasoconstrictor, _____ is produced when the renin–aldosterone–angiotensin system (RAAS) is activated.

2. The _____ is defined as the volume of blood ejected from the left ventricle in 1 minute.

3. _____ is defined as resistance to the flow of blood in peripheral arterial vessels that is associated with blood vessel diameter, vessel length, and blood viscosity.

4. _____ is the measure of blood pressure when the heart is at rest (diastole).

5. The term for increased sensitivity to sun exposure that can result in sunburn is _____.

6. _____ is a hormone that promotes sodium and fluid reabsorption.

7. The term for deficient serum potassium levels is _____.

8. The term for elevated diastolic or systolic blood pressure is _____.

9. _____ is the measure of the pressure when the heart's ventricles are contracting (systole).

10. A sudden drop in blood pressure that occurs when arising from lying down or sitting to standing is called

   _____.

11. The term for excessive serum potassium levels is _____.

12. _____ is the name of the enzyme that catalyzes the conversion of angiotensin I to angiotensin II.

13. _____ is defined as systolic blood pressure ranging between 120 and 139 mm Hg and diastolic blood pressure ranging between 80 and 89 mm Hg.

14. The _____ is activated when there is a drop in renal blood flow that increases blood volume, blood flow to the kidney, vasoconstriction, and blood pressure.

15. _____ is a drug that produces diuresis (urination).

16. _____ is nighttime urination.

17. _____ is painful breast enlargement in men.

18. _____ is increased uric acid levels in the blood that is produced by some diuretics and can aggravate gout.

19. _____ is excessive hair growth in women.

20. _____ is a sudden rise in blood pressure, excessive weight gain, generalized edema, proteinuria, severe headache, and visual disturbances occurring in late pregnancy.

21. _____ is a measure of human body size and proportion. It is defined as the weight in kilograms divided by the square of the height in meters.

22. _____ is the elevated systolic blood pressure only. Diastolic blood pressure is within the normal range.

23. _____ is characterized by excessive serum sodium levels.

24. _____ is an important risk factor of hypertension that promotes the development of atherosclerosis and cardiovascular disease.

25. _____ is characterized by deficient serum sodium levels.

MULTIPLE CHOICE

1. The formula for calculating blood pressure is

   _____.
   A. $BP = HR \times CO$
   B. $BP = HR \times PR$
   C. $BP = CO \times NaCl$
   D. $BP = CO \times PR$

2. Ca^{2+} channel blockers may used in the treatment of

   _____.
   A. angina only
   B. hypertension only
   C. angina and hypertension

3. Which of the following effects of Ca^{2+} channel blockers is responsible for reducing blood pressure?

   _____
   A. increased force of cardiac contractions leading to increased cardiac output
   B. relaxation of blood vessels (decreased peripheral resistance)
   C. decreased renal blood flow
   D. increased heart rate

4. Diastolic hypertension is the predominant form of

   hypertension before age _____.
   A. 50 years
   B. 60 years
   C. 70 years
   D. 80 years

5. Stage 1 hypertension is classified as systolic blood

   pressure ranges between _____.
   A. 100 to 120 mm Hg systolic and 70 to 80 mm Hg diastolic
   B. 120 to 139 mm Hg systolic and 80 to 89 mm Hg diastolic
   C. 140 to 159 mm Hg systolic and 90 to 99 mm Hg diastolic
   D. $\geq$160 mm Hg systolic and $\geq$100 mm Hg diastolic

6. All of the following are classifications for diuretics

   except _____.
   A. thiazides
   B. loop
   C. calcium sparing
   D. potassium sparing

7. Pharmacy technicians should apply the warning label

   _____ to prescription vials containing potassium-sparing diuretics.
   A. MAY BE ADVISABLE TO EAT BANANAS OR DRINK ORANGE JUICE
   B. AVOID SALT SUBSTITUTES
   C. MAY CAUSE DROWSINESS
   D. TAKE WITH LOTS OF WATER

8. Select the **false** statement about ACE inhibitors.

   _____
   A. ACE inhibitors block the conversion of angiotensin I to angiotensin II (a potent vasoconstrictor).
   B. Dry cough is a common side effect of ACE inhibitors.
   C. ACE inhibitors produce potassium loss.
   D. ACE inhibitors are contraindicated in pregnancy because they can interfere with fetal development of the kidneys.

9. Select the **false** statement about beta blockers.

   _____
   A. Beta blockers lower blood pressure by increasing heart rate.
   B. Beta blockers decrease peripheral resistance.
   C. Beta blockers used in the treatment of hypertension may be selective (β_1) or nonselective (β_1, β_2).
   D. Beta blockers are contraindicated in asthma and diabetes.

10. Select the pair of angiotensin II antagonists.

   _____
   A. Coreg and Trandate
   B. Prinivil and Vasotec
   C. Inderal and Tenormin
   D. Cozaar and Diovan

FILL IN THE BLANK: DRUG NAMES

1. What is the *brand name* for hydrochlorothiazide (HCTZ)? _____

2. What is the *generic name* for Lasix? _____

3. What is the *brand name* for spironolactone? _____

4. What is the *generic name* for Lotensin? _____

5. What is the *brand name* for captopril? _____

6. What is the *generic name* for Vasotec? _____

7. What are two *brand names* for lisinopril? _____

8. What is the *generic name* for Altace? _____

9. What are two *brand name*s for lisinopril plus hydrochlorothiazide? _____

10. What is the *generic name* for Cozaar? _____

11. What is the *brand name* for valsartan? _____

12. What is the *generic name* for Hyzaar? _____

13. What is the *brand name* for valsartan plus hydrochlorothiazide? _____

MATCHING

Match each drug to its pharmacological classification.

1. _____ spironolactone 25 mg   A. thiazide diuretic

2. _____ benazepril 10 mg   B. ACE inhibitor

3. _____ nadolol 40 mg   C. angiotensin II antagonist

4. _____ eprosartan 400 mg   D. beta blocker

5. _____ indapamide 1.25 mg   E. aldosterone receptor blocker

MATCHING

Match each drug to its pharmacological classification.

1. _____ bisoprolol 10 mg   A. thiazide diuretic

2. _____ Vasotec 2.5 mg   B. ACE inhibitor

3. _____ furosemide 40 mg   C. angiotensin II antagonist

4. _____ chlorthalidone 50 mg   D. beta blocker

5. _____ losartan 25 mg   E. loop diuretic

MATCHING

Match each drug to its pharmacological classification.

1. _____ Monopril 20 mg   A. potassium-sparing diuretic

2. _____ carvedilol 6.25 mg   B. combined alpha and beta blocker

3. _____ nadolol 40 mg   C. α_1-antagonists

4. _____ triamterene plus HCTZ 37.5 mg/75 mg   D. ACE inhibitor

5. _____ doxazosin 1 mg   E. beta blocker

MATCHING

Patient education is an essential component of therapeutics. Select the **best** warning label to apply to the prescription vial given to patients taking the drugs listed.

1. _____ Inderal LA 120 mg   A. MAY BE ADVISABLE TO EAT BANANAS OR DRINK ORANGE JUICE

2. _____ amiloride plus HCTZ

3. _____ captopril 12.5 mg   B. TAKE WITH FOOD

4. _____ bumetanide 1 mg   C. MAY CAUSE A DRY COUGH

5. _____ spironolactone 25 mg   D. DON'T CRUSH OR CHEW

     E. AVOID PROLONGED EXPOSURE TO SUNLIGHT

MATCHING

Patient education is an essential component of therapeutics. Select the **best** warning label to apply to the prescription vial given to patients taking the drugs listed.

1. _____ metoprolol SR 100 mg   A. ROTATE SITE OF APPLICATION

2. _____ clonidine 0.1 mg patch   B. AVOID PREGNANCY

3. _____ ramipril 10 mg   C. MAY BE ADVISABLE TO EAT BANANAS OR DRINK ORANGE JUICE

4. _____ valsartan

5. _____ furosemide 20 mg   D. AVOID SALT SUBSTITUTES AND POTASSIUM RICH DIETS

     E. DON'T CRUSH OR CHEW

TRUE OR FALSE

1. _____ Complications of untreated hypertension include stroke, myocardial infarction, and kidney damage.

2. _____ Lifestyle factors that increase the risk for hypertension are tobacco use, decreased physical activity, diets high in salt and saturated fats, and excessive alcohol consumption.

3. _____ The normal average blood pressure is 140/90 mm Hg.

4. _____ Sites for blood pressure control are the kidneys, heart, blood vessels, and lungs.

5. _____ When peripheral vascular resistance increases, blood pressure increases.

6. _____ Metabolic syndrome reduces the development of atherosclerosis and cardiovascular disease.

7. _____ Hydralazine is recommended for hypertensive emergencies (parenteral use) and is safe for use in pregnant women.

CRITICAL THINKING

The following hard copies are brought to your pharmacy for filling. Identify the prescription error(s). (You already have the patient's full address on file.)

```
┌─────────────────────────────────────────┐
│        Anh Dang Tu, MD      Date _____ │
│        1145 Broadway                     │
│        Anytown, USA                      │
│                                          │
│ Pt. Name _____ Lili Olschefsky _____│
│ Address _____│
│ Rx   Trandate 200mg tablet    #30        │
│        i QID                             │
│                                          │
│                                          │
│ Refills _____                          │
│                                          │
│ _____        Tu         │
│ _____    _____ │
│ Substitution permitted    Dispense as written │
└─────────────────────────────────────────┘
```

1. Spot the error in the following prescription:

   _____

   A. Quantity missing
   B. Strength missing
   C. Directions missing
   D. Directions incorrect
   E. Dosage form incorrect

```
┌─────────────────────────────────────────┐
│        Kathy Principi, MD    Date _____│
│        1145 Broadway                     │
│        Anytown, USA                      │
│                                          │
│ Pt. Name _____ Will Jones _____│
│ Address _____│
│ Rx   Prinizide    #30                    │
│        1-2 tablets daily                 │
│                                          │
│ Refills _____                          │
│       Principi                           │
│ _____        _____ │
│ Substitution permitted    Dispense as written │
└─────────────────────────────────────────┘
```

2. Spot the error in the following prescription:

   _____

   A. Quantity missing
   B. Directions missing
   C. Strength missing
   D. Directions incorrect
   E. Dosage form incorrect

```
        Kathy Principi, MD       Date _____
            1145 Broadway
            Anytown, USA
Pt. Name _____ Ellen Wilber _____
Address _____

Rx   Capoten 50mg capsule    #60
        i BID


Refills _____
____ Principi _____    _____
Substitution permitted    Dispense as written
```

3. Spot the error in the following prescription:

   _____

   A. Quantity missing
   B. Strength missing
   C. Directions missing
   D. Directions incorrect
   E. Dosage form incorrect

```
        Kathy Principi, MD       Date _____
            1145 Broadway
            Anytown, USA
Pt. Name _____ Preston Scott _____
Address _____

Rx   nifedipine 60mg XL    #30
        ss tab QD


Refills _____
____ Principi _____    _____
Substitution permitted    Dispense as written
```

4. Spot the error in the following prescription:

   _____

   A. Quantity missing
   B. Strength missing
   C. Directions missing
   D. Directions incorrect
   E. Dosage form incorrect

5. Give six pairs of drug names that have look-alike or sound-alike issues with drugs used to treat migraine headache or treat hypertension.

DRUG NAME	LOOK-ALIKE OR SOUND-ALIKE DRUG

6. Write a short paragraph **describing the relationship** between the kidneys and blood pressure control. List three classes of medication that have the kidney as their site of action.

_____

_____

_____

_____

_____

RESEARCH ACTIVITY

Access the National Library of Medicine's Website (http://www.nlm.nih.gov/medlineplus/highbloodpressure.html) to answer the following questions.

1. Why is hypertension classified as a chronic disease of lifestyle?

_____

_____

_____

_____

_____

2. What lifestyle changes are recommended?

_____

_____

_____

_____

_____

23 Treatment of Heart Failure

TERMS AND DEFINITIONS

Match each term with the correct definition below. Some terms may not be used.

A. Automaticity

B. Cardioglycosides

C. Digitalization

D. Ejection fraction

E. Heart failure

F. Natriuretic peptides

G. Positive inotropic effect

H. Stroke volume

1. The _____ are a class of drugs, most commonly derived from foxglove, that have the ability to alter cardiovascular function.

2. _____ is the process of rapidly increasing the initial dose of digoxin until the therapeutic dose is achieved.

3. _____ is equal to the volume of blood ejected by the left ventricle during each cardiac contraction minus the volume of blood in the ventricle at the end of systole.

4. _____ is a clinical syndrome in which the heart is unable to pump blood at a rate to meet the body's metabolic needs.

5. The spontaneous depolarization (contraction) of heart cells is called _____.

6. _____ are hormones that play a role in cardiac homeostasis.

7. The percentage of blood ejected from the left ventricle with each heartbeat is called the _____.

8. An increase in the force of myocardial contractions is known as a(n) _____.

MULTIPLE CHOICE

1. Drugs used in the treatment of heart failure include

   _____.
   A. digoxin
   B. hydrochlorothiazide
   C. lisinopril
   D. metoprolol
   E. all of the above

2. Persons with stage B heart failure have

   _____.
   A. a high risk for developing heart failure
   B. structural changes without symptoms
   C. advanced structural heart disease plus heart failure symptoms

3. Regarding compensatory mechanisms that are "switched on" when the heart function fails, all of the following statements are true *except*

   _____.
   A. the renin–aldosterone–angiotensin system is activated to increase blood volume.
   B. the renin–aldosterone–angiotensin system is activated to increase cardiac output.
   C. natriuretic peptides (hormones) are released to promote vasoconstriction.
   D. natriuretic peptides (hormones) are released to promote sodium and water elimination by the kidneys.

4. Digitalis is a cardioglycoside derived from

   _____.
   A. foxglove
   B. mushroom
   C. cinchona bark
   D. poppy

5. Which statement about digoxin is *true*?

   _____.
   A. It decreases the force of myocardial contractions.
   B. It decreases exercise tolerance.
   C. It increases the force of myocardial contractions.
   D. It decreases cardiac output.

6. Select the *false* statement. Digoxin should be

   administered along with _____.
   A. ACE inhibitors
   B. beta blockers
   C. diuretics
   D. calcium channel blockers

7. Pharmacy technicians should apply the warning

   label _____ to prescription vials containing digoxin:
   A. MAY BE ADVISABLE TO EAT BANANAS OR DRINK ORANGE JUICE
   B. TAKE AS DIRECTED; DON'T SKIP OR EXCEED DOSAGE
   C. TAKE WITH LOTS OF WATER
   D. AVOID PROLONGED EXPOSURE TO SUNLIGHT

8. An antidote for digoxin toxicity is

   _____.
   A. Digibind
   B. Lanoxin
   C. Digitek
   D. Lanoxicap

9. All of the following drugs are used in the treatment

   of heart failure *except* _____.
   A. angiotensin II receptor antagonists
   B. "statins"
   C. vasodilators
   D. NSAIDs

10. Digoxin is available in all of the dosage forms

   except _____.
   A. transdermal patch
   B. capsule
   C. tablet
   D. elixir
   E. injection

FILL IN THE BLANK: DRUG NAMES

1. What is the ***generic name*** for Lanoxin? _____

2. What is the ***brand name*** for chlorothiazide? _____

3. What is the ***generic name*** for Thalitone? _____

4. What is the ***brand name*** for hydrochlorothiazide? _____

5. What is the *generic name* for Lozol (United States) and Lozide (Canada)? _____

6. What is the *generic name* for Bumex (United States) and Burinex (Canada)? _____

7. What is the *brand name* for furosemide? _____

8. What is the *generic name* for Aldactone? _____

9. What is the *generic name* for Zebeta (United States) and Monocor (Canada)? _____

10. What is the *generic name* for Toprol XL (United States) and Lopressor SR (Canada)? _____

11. What is the *brand name* for carvedilol? _____

12. What is the *brand name* for benazepril? _____

13. What is the *brand name* for captopril? _____

14. What is the *brand name* for enalapril? _____

15. What is the *generic name* for Prinivil and Zestril? _____

16. What is the *brand name* for quinapril? _____

17. What is the *generic name* for Altace? _____

18. What is the *brand name* for candesartan? _____

19. What is the *generic name* for Cozaar? _____

20. What is the *brand name* for valsartan? _____

21. What is the *generic name* for Apresoline? _____

22. What is the *brand name* for isosorbide dinitrate? _____

MATCHING

Match each drug to its pharmacological classification. (Classifications can be used more than once.)

1. _____ carvedilol 6.25 mg

2. _____ digoxin 0.25 mg

3. _____ benazepril 10 mg

4. _____ eprosartan 400 mg

5. _____ indapamide 1.25 mg

A. thiazide diuretic

B. ACE inhibitor

C. angiotensin II antagonist

D. combined alpha and beta blockers

E. cardioglycoside

MATCHING

Match each drug to its pharmacological classification.

1. _____ furosemide 20 mg

2. _____ Vasotec 2.5 mg

3. _____ chlorthalidone 50 mg

4. _____ losartan 25 mg

A. thiazide diuretic

B. ACE inhibitor

C. angiotensin II antagonist

D. loop diuretic

MATCHING

Match each drug to its pharmacological classification.

1. _____ Bumex 0.5 mg

2. _____ hydralazine 25 mg

3. _____ Digibind 30 mg

4. _____ Lopressor 25 mg

5. _____ Hyzaar 50-12.5 mg

A. vasodilators

B. digoxin antidote

C. beta blocker

D. loop diuretic

E. angiotensin II antagonist plus diuretic

MATCHING

Patient education is an essential component of therapeutics. Select the **best** warning label to apply to the prescription vial given to patients taking the drugs listed.

1. _____ Inderal LA 120 mg

2. _____ valsartan 40 mg

3. _____ bumetanide 1 mg

4. _____ spironolactone 25 mg

5. _____ isosorbide dinitrate 5 mg

A. AVOID PREGNANCY

B. TAKE WITH FOOD

C. TAKE ON AN EMPTY STOMACH

D. SWALLOW WHOLE: DON'T CRUSH OR CHEW

E. AVOID PROLONGED EXPOSURE TO SUNLIGHT

TRUE OR FALSE

1. _____ Heart failure may affect the left side of the heart, the right side of the heart, or both sides.

2. _____ Lifestyle factors that worsen heart failure are decreased physical activity, diets high in salt and saturated fats, and excessive alcohol consumption.

3. _____ There are two stages of heart failure.

4. _____ The bioavailability of digoxin differs between commercial manufacturers.

5. _____ Food can increase the absorption of digoxin.

6. _____ Nonsteroidal anti-inflammatory drugs worsen edema and interfere with the effect of drugs used to treat heart failure such as ACE inhibitors.

7. _____ Digoxin should be prescribed to women with heart failure to decrease the risk for mortality.

CRITICAL THINKING

The following hard copies are brought to your pharmacy for filling. Identify the prescription error(s). (You already have the patient's full address on file.)

```
Kathy Principi, MD        Date _____
1145 Broadway
Anytown, USA

Pt. Name _____ Bill Carey _____
Address _____

R      digoxin tablet      #30
       1 tablet QD



Refills _____
____Principi_____    _____
Substitution permitted        Dispense as written
```

1. Spot the error in the following prescription:

   _____

   A. Quantity missing
   B. Directions incomplete
   C. Strength missing
   D. Strength incorrect
   E. Dosage form incorrect

```
Marc Cordova, MD         Date _____
1145 Broadway
Anytown, USA

Pt. Name _____ Bill Carey _____
Address _____

R   Hydralazine 2.5mg     #60      i BID
    isosorbide dinitrate 5mg   #60    i BID



Refills _____
____Cordova_____    _____
Substitution permitted        Dispense as written
```

2. Spot the error in the following prescription:

   _____

   A. Quantity missing
   B. Directions incomplete
   C. Strength missing
   D. Strength incorrect
   E. Dosage form incorrect

```
Kathy Principi, MD        Date _____
1145 Broadway
Anytown, USA

Pt. Name _____ Ellen Wilber _____
Address _____

R   metoprolol extended release 100mg tab
    i QD



Refills _____
____Principi_____    _____
Substitution permitted        Dispense as written
```

3. Spot the error in the following prescription:

   _____

   A. Quantity missing
   B. Directions incomplete
   C. Strength missing
   D. Strength incorrect
   E. Dosage form incorrect

```
┌─────────────────────────────────────────┐
│         Kathy Principi, MD    Date _____ │
│            1145 Broadway                  │
│            Anytown, USA                   │
│                                           │
│  Pt. Name _____ Will Jones _____  │
│  Address _____  │
│                                           │
│  ℞   bumetanide    #30                    │
│         1 tablet daily                    │
│                                           │
│                                           │
│  Refills _____                           │
│  ____Principi_____   _____   │
│  Substitution permitted   Dispense as written │
└─────────────────────────────────────────┘
```

4. Spot the error in the following prescription:

   _____

   A. Quantity missing
   B. Directions incomplete
   C. Strength missing
   D. Strength incorrect
   E. Dosage form incorrect

```
┌─────────────────────────────────────────┐
│         Kathy Principi, MD    Date _____ │
│            1145 Broadway                  │
│            Anytown, USA                   │
│                                           │
│  Pt. Name _____ Ellen Wilber _____  │
│  Address _____  │
│                                           │
│  ℞   carvedilol 25mg BID    #60 capsules  │
│                                           │
│                                           │
│  Refills _____                           │
│  ____Principi_____   _____   │
│  Substitution permitted   Dispense as written │
└─────────────────────────────────────────┘
```

5. Spot the error in the following prescription:

   _____

   A. Quantity missing
   B. Directions incomplete
   C. Strength missing
   D. Strength incorrect
   E. Dosage form incorrect

6. Samuel Carlson, age 5 years, takes digoxin 0.125 mg PO daily. Digoxin comes in liquid form. The elixir is supplied as 0.05 mg/mL. How many milliliters will Samuel need to take to get 0.125 mg of digoxin?

_____

_____

_____

_____

_____

RESEARCH ACTIVITY

Access the National Library of Medicine's website (http://www.nhlbi.nih.gov/health/dci/Diseases/Hf/HF_WhatIs.html) to answer the following questions.

1. Why is lifestyle change a key component in the treatment of heart failure?

_____

_____

_____

_____

_____

2. Make a list of lifestyle changes that are recommended.

_____

_____

_____

_____

_____

RESEARCH ACTIVITY

1. Review the patient profile below and answer the questions.

Last name: Petrosky   First name: Joe   Gender: M

Address: 1906 E Denny Wy   Anytown, USA 98122   BD: 040346

Allergies: penicillin

Comment: $8/12 copay   Disc.:   Phone: 206-322-6789

Ins: PC Plan: 05   Group#:12345678   ID#: 526458904

Copay: $8.00

Cardholder: Petrosky   Joe   Exp. date: 12-31-08

DATE	RX#	DRUG AND STRENGTH	SIG	QTY	MD	RF
1-2-08	72345	bumetanide 1 mg	1 QD	100	Johnson, C	2
2-4-08	79278	Cardizem 180 mg CD	1 QD	60	Johnson	1
3-1-08	81956	Cotrim DS	1 BID	20	Principi, K	
3-1-08	84358	naproxen 550 mg	1 BID	120	Principi, K	
3-2-08	72345	bumetanide 1 mg	1 QD	100	Johnson, C	1
3-4-08	79278	Cardizem 180 mg CD	1 QD	60	Johnson	1
3-16-08	96346	lisinopril 10 mg	1 BID	60	Johnson	2
3-30-08	102344	digoxin 0.25 mg	1 QD	30	Johnson	4
4-12-08	96346	lisinopril 10 mg	1 BID	60	Johnson	1
4-30-08	102344	digoxin 0.25 mg	1 QD	30	Johnson	4
5-4-08	105278	Rhythmol 150 mg	1 Q8h	90	Johnson	1
5-30-08	102344	digoxin 0.25 mg	1 QD	30	Johnson	3

A. Joe Petrosky brings in a renewal prescription for lisinopril. Lisinopril is manufactured by two companies. Develop a list of questions you might ask to identify the manufacturer's product he previously received.

_____

_____

_____

_____

_____

B. Review Mr. Petrosky's patient profile. Make a list of the medication he takes that are used in the treatment of CHF.

_____

_____

_____

_____

_____

C. Explain why each of these classes of medication might be used for the treatment of CHF.

_____

_____

_____

_____

_____

24 Treatment of Myocardial Infarction and Stroke

TERMS AND DEFINITIONS

Match each term with the correct definition below. Some terms may not be used.

A. Infarction

B. High-density lipoproteins (HDLs)

C. Triglycerides

D. Low-density lipoproteins (LDLs)

E. Partial thromboplastin time (PTT)

F. Prothrombin time (PT)

G. Stenosis

H. Thrombosis

I. Transient ischemic attack (TIA)

J. Anticoagulant

K. Antiplatelet drug

L. Antithrombotic

M. Cholesterol

N. Hemorrhagic stroke

O. Aneurysm

P. Anoxia

Q. Atherosclerosis

R. Atherothrombosis

S. Embolic stroke

T. Hemostasis

U. Hypoxia

V. Ischemia

W. Ischemic stroke

X. Lipoprotein

Y. Mitral valve stenosis

Z. Necrosis

AA. Plaque

BB. Platelets

CC. Rhabdomyolysis

DD. Thrombolytic

EE. Thrombolytic stroke

1. A sudden loss of blood supply that results in cell death is known as a(n) _____.

2. A stroke caused by an emboli obstructing the flow of blood through an artery is known as a(n)

   _____.

3. High-density lipoproteins (HDLs) are also known as _____.

4. Low-density lipoproteins (LDLs) are also known as _____.

5. _____ is a test given to determine effectiveness of heparin in reducing antithrombotic activity.

6. _____ is a test given to determine the effectiveness of warfarin in reducing clotting time.

7. The stiffening and narrowing of artery walls is called _____.

8. The formation of a blood clot is called _____.

9. A stroke that typically lasts for only a few minutes is called _____.

10. Sudden bleeding into or around the brain may cause a(n) _____.

11. A(n) _____ is a drug that prolongs coagulation time and is used to prevent clot formation.

12. A(n) _____ is a drug that prevents accumulation of platelets, thereby blocking an important step in the clot formation process.

13. A(n) _____ is a drug that inhibits clot formation by reducing the coagulation action of the blood protein thrombin.

14. _____ is a naturally occurring, waxy substance produced by the liver and found in foods that maintains cell membranes and is needed for vitamin D production.

15. _____ is the process of stopping the flow of blood.

16. _____ is the reduced oxygen delivery to the cells.

17. Ischemia in the brain is known as _____.

18. _____ is a weakened spot of the artery wall that has stretched or burst, filling the area with blood and causing damage.

19. _____ is the disease of the mitral valve involving buildup of plaque-like material around the valve.

20. Small globules of cholesterol covered by a layer of protein is known as _____.

21. _____ is known as cell death.

22. _____ are the storage forms of energy found in fat tissue muscle.

23. Fatty cholesterol deposits are known as _____.

24. Formation of a blood clot in an artery is known as _____.

25. _____ is the absence of oxygen supply to cells that results in cell damage or death.

26. _____ is known as the build up of lipids and plaque inside artery walls, impeding the flow of blood and oxygen.

27. _____ is a stroke caused by thrombosis.

28. The reduction of blood supplied to tissues that is typically caused by blood vessel obstruction from atherosclerosis, stenosis, or plaque is known as _____.

29. _____ are structures found in the blood that are involved in the coagulation process.

30. The breakdown of muscle fibers and release of muscle fiber contents into the circulation is known as _____.

31. _____ is a drug used to dissolve blood clots.

MULTIPLE CHOICE

1. Drugs used in the treatment of myocardial infarction and stroke include all of the following *except* _____.
   A. digoxin
   B. Lipitor
   C. rosuvastatin
   D. warfarin
   E. clopidogrel

2. MI and stroke may be caused by _____.
   A. chronic inflammation of arteries that supply the heart and brain
   B. atherosclerosis
   C. atherothrombosis
   D. all of the above

3. Thrombolytics are derived from _____.
   A. recombinant DNA
   B. bacterial cultures (streptococci)
   C. kidney cell extracts
   D. human tissue plasminogen activator
   E. all of the above

4. Modifiable risk factors are _____.
   A. smoking and heavy alcohol consumption
   B. family history
   C. diet high in cholesterol
   D. age and gender
   E. A and C

5. Select the **false** answer about drugs used to control hemostasis. _____
   A. Anticoagulants promote coagulation.
   B. Antiplatelet drugs interfere with early steps in the clot formation process.
   C. Fibrinolytics (thrombolytics) dissolve existing clots.
   D. Anticoagulants lessen coagulation.

6. Select the class of drug that is *not* used in the treatment of MI and stroke. _____
   A. anticoagulant drugs
   B. antiplatelet drugs
   C. ACE inhibitors
   D. antihyperlipidemics
   E. thrombolytics

7. Select the antiplatelet drug that must be administered

   parenterally. _____
   A. aspirin
   B. abciximab
   C. clopidogrel
   D. ticlopidine
   E. dipyridamole

8. Warfarin interferes with the formation of

   _____ clotting factors.
   A. vitamin A–dependent
   B. vitamin E–dependent
   C. vitamin D–dependent
   D. vitamin K–dependent

9. The antidote for warfarin overdose is

   _____.
   A. heparin
   B. vitamin K
   C. Coumadin
   D. vitamin D

10. The antidote for heparin overdose is

   _____.
   A. vitamin K
   B. protamine zinc
   C. protamine sulfate
   D. vitamin D

FILL IN THE BLANK: DRUG NAMES

1. What is the *generic name* for Plavix? _____

2. What is the *brand name* for dipyridamole? _____

3. What is the *generic name* for Ticlid? _____

4. What is the *brand name* for dipyridamole plus aspirin? _____

5. What is the *generic name* for Coumadin? _____

6. What is the *brand name* for dalteparin? _____

7. What is the *generic name* for Lovenox? _____

8. What a *brand name* for heparin sodium? _____

9. What is the *generic name* for Innohep? _____

10. What is the *brand name* for alteplase? _____

11. What is the *generic name* for Streptase (Canada)? _____

12. What is the *brand name* for tenecteplase? _____

13. What is the *generic name* for Lipitor? _____

14. What is the *brand name* for fluvastatin? _____

15. What is the *generic name* for Mevacor? _____

16. What is the *brand name* for pravastatin? _____

17. What is the *generic name* for Crestor? _____

18. What is the *brand name* for simvastatin? _____

19. What is the *generic name* for Vytorin (United States)? _____

20. What is the *brand name* for aspirin plus pravastatin? _____

21. What is the *generic name* for Caduet? _____

22. What is the *brand name* for niacin plus lovastatin? _____

23. What is the *generic name* for Lopid? _____

24. What is the *generic name* for Tricor (United States) and Lipidil (Canada)? _____

25. What is the *brand name* for colestipol? _____

26. What is the *brand name* for niacin? _____

MATCHING

Patient education is an essential component of therapeutics. Select the **best** warning label to apply to the prescription vial given to patients taking the drugs listed.

1. _____ Aggrenox 25 to 200 mg   A. AVOID GRAPEFRUIT JUICE

2. _____ warfarin 2 mg   B. SWALLOW WHOLE; DO NOT CRUSH OR CHEW

3. _____ cholestyramine 4 g   C. AVOID PREGNANCY

4. _____ Lipitor 20 mg   D. TAKE 1 HOUR BEFORE OR 4 HOURS AFTER OTHER DRUGS

MATCHING

Patient education is an essential component of therapeutics. Select the **best** warning label to apply to the prescription vial given to patients taking the drugs listed.

1. _____ niacin   A. TAKE ON AN EMPTY STOMACH

2. _____ Zocor 10 mg   B. TAKE WITH FOOD

3. _____ gemfibrozil 600 mg   C. SWALLOW WHOLE; DON'T CRUSH OR CHEW

4. _____ Welchol   D. AVOID GRAPEFRUIT JUICE

                                        E. AVOID PREGNANCY

MATCHING

Match each drug to its pharmacological classification. (Classifications may be used more than once.)

1. _____ Lovenox

2. _____ streptokinase

3. _____ rosuvastatin

4. _____ clopidogrel

5. _____ simvastatin

6. _____ dipyridamole

7. _____ alteplase

8. _____ heparin

9. _____ Lescol

10. _____ cholestyramine

11. _____ abciximab

12. _____ Tricor

13. _____ warfarin

14. _____ lovastatin

A. antiplatelet

B. thrombolytic

C. antihyperlipidemic

D. anticoagulant

TRUE OR FALSE

1. _____ Prothrombin time (PT) test is also known as Pro-Time, INR test.

2. _____ A transient ischemic attack (TIA) is also known as a mini-stroke.

3. _____ Atherosclerosis is caused by too little LDL in the blood.

4. _____ Symptoms of a myocardial infarction last 1 to 5 minutes and may be relieved by rest.

5. _____ Myocardial infarction is the leading cause of death in the United States.

6. _____ Myocardial infarction produces symptoms that are similar to those of angina.

7. _____ Drugs administered to prevent stroke and myocardial infarction may be administered to control the buildup of lipids and plaque and reduce the formation of blood clots.

8. _____ Low-molecular-weight heparins are substitutable.

CRITICAL THINKING

The following hard copies are brought to your pharmacy for filling. Identify the prescription error. (You already have the patient's full address on file.)

Harry S. Lo
1247 S Jackson St
Anytown, USA 98104

Date _5-31-08_

Pt. Name _____ Michiko Nagawa _____

Address _____

℞ atorvastatin 20mg tablet
       i QD

Refills _____

_____ H. Lo _____

Substitution permitted   Dispense as written

---

1. Spot the error in the following prescription:

   _____

   A. Quantity missing
   B. Directions missing
   C. Strength missing
   D. Directions incorrect
   E. Dosage form incorrect

Marc Cordova, MD
1145 Broadway
Anytown, USA

Date _5-20-08_

Pt. Name _____ Bill Carey _____

Address _____

℞ Plavix 75mg tablet #60
       i tablet QID daily

Refills _____

_____ Cordova _____

Substitution permitted   Dispense as written

---

2. Spot the error in the following prescription:

   _____

   A. Quantity missing
   B. Directions missing
   C. Strength missing
   D. Directions incorrect
   E. Dosage form incorrect

Kathy Principi, MD
1145 Broadway
Anytown, USA

Date _5-22-08_

Pt. Name _____ Ellen Wilber _____

Address _____

℞ Coumadin 5mg tab #30 i QD
     ibuprofen 800mg tab #30 1 TID prn

Refills _____

_____ Principi _____

Substitution permitted   Dispense as written

---

3. Spot the error in the following prescription:

   _____

   A. Quantity missing
   B. Strength missing
   C. Directions missing
   D. Drug interaction
   E. Dosage form incorrect

4. Mr. Cowan has recently had a myocardial infarction and heparin is ordered. You must prepare an IV containing heparin 42,000 units in 1 L of D5NS. He is to receive 25 mL/hr. How many units of heparin will he receive per hour?

_____

_____

_____

_____

_____

5. Mr. Cowan is discharged early, and Lovenox 40 mg SC daily is prescribed. The pharmacy stocks 300-mg/3-mL multidose vials. How many doses are in one vial?

_____

_____

_____

_____

_____

6. You are instructed to prepare alteplase for a recently admitted stroke patient. The usual dose is 15 mg IV bolus followed by 50 mg infused over 30 minutes and then 35 mg infused over 60 minutes. If alteplase (Activase) powder for injection comes in two size vials—50 mg (29 million IU) and 100 mg (58 million IU)—which vial should be selected for the complete course of therapy if only ONE vial is to be reconstituted?

_____

_____

_____

_____

_____

RESEARCH ACTIVITY

1. "Take aspirin daily and stop smoking cigarettes" is advice given to patients who have had a stroke or myocardial infarction. Why are these recommendations made? Conduct an Internet search to answer the question. You may begin your search by visiting http://www.nlm.nih.gov/medlineplus/tutorials/preventingstrokes/hp139102.pdf and http://circ.ahajournals.org/cgi/content/full/96/8/2751.

_____

_____

_____

_____

_____

25 Treatment of Arrhythmia

TERMS AND DEFINITIONS

Match each term with the correct definition below. Some terms may not be used.

A. Atrial fibrillation

B. Atrial flutter

C. Automaticity

D. Ectopic

E. Electrical cardioversion

F. Refractory period

G. Repolarization

H. Supraventricular tachycardia

I. Ventricular tachycardia

J. Ventricular fibrillation

K. Depolarization

1. The _____ is the time between contractions that it takes for repolarization to occur.

2. During _____, the atria beat between 300 and 400 beats/min, and contractions are uncoordinated.

3. The period of time when the heart is recharging and preparing for another contraction is called _____.

4. A(n) _____ beat is a heartbeat that occurs outside of the normal pacemaker locations.

5. Persons who have a(n) _____ have a heart rate of 160 to 350 beats per min and contractions of the atrium exceed the number in the ventricles.

6. The term used to describe spontaneous contraction of heart muscle cells is _____.

7. _____ is the process of applying an electrical shock to the heart with a defibrillator.

8. An arrhythmia that produces heartbeats up to 600 beats/min and uncoordinated contractions is _____.

9. _____ occurs in a region above the ventricles and produces a heart rate up to 200 beats/min.

10. _____ causes the ventricles to beat faster than 200 beats/min.

11. _____ is the process where the heart muscle conducts an electrical impulse, causing a contraction.

MULTIPLE CHOICE

1. The process where the heart muscle conducts an electrical impulse causing a contraction is called

   _____.
   A. repolarization
   B. depolarization
   C. automaticity
   D. refractory period

2. _____ is a life-threatening arrhythmia in which the heart beats more rapidly than in all other arrhythmias.
   A. Atrial fibrillation
   B. Atrial flutter
   C. Ventricular tachycardia
   D. Ventricular fibrillation

3. Supraventricular tachycardia is an arrhythmia that

   originates in an area _____ the ventricles.
   A. below
   B. above
   C. within

4. Select the nonmodifiable risk factor for arrhythmia.

   _____
   A. Obesity
   B. Age
   C. Smoking
   D. Excessive alcohol consumption
   E. Stimulant use

5. Which of the following is *not* a disease risk factor for

   arrhythmia? _____
   A. Coronary heart disease (CHD) and stroke
   B. Diabetes
   C. Thyroid disease
   D. Obstructive sleep apnea
   E. Epilepsy

6. Digoxin is approved for the treatment of

   _____.
   A. atrial fibrillation
   B. ventricular fibrillation
   C. ventricular tachycardia
   D. supraventricular tachycardia

7. _____ and _____ can significantly reduce the risk for first-time atrial fibrillation in patients with hypertension and heart failure and after myocardial infarction.
   A. Nitrates and diuretics
   B. ACE inhibitors and ARBs
   C. Diuretics and calcium channel blockers
   D. Nitrates and cholinergics

8. Tinnitus is a sign of _____ toxicity.
   A. amiodarone
   B. procainamide
   C. mexiletine
   D. quinidine

9. Which class I antiarrhythmic drug must be adminis-

   tered parenterally? _____
   A. procainamide
   B. lidocaine
   C. tocainide
   D. propafenone

10. Persons taking amiodarone may experience all of the following adverse effects *except*

    _____.
    A. constipation
    B. photosensitivity
    C. skin discoloration
    D. visual disturbances
    E. corneal deposits

FILL IN THE BLANK: DRUG NAMES

1. What is the **brand name** for flecainide? _____

2. What is the **generic name** for Norpace (United States) and Rythmodan (Canada)? _____

3. What is a **brand name** for propafenone? _____

4. What is the **generic name** for Pronestyl SR (United States) and Procan SR (Canada)? _____

5. What is the **generic name** for Quinadure (United States)? _____

6. What is the **brand name** for acebutolol? _____

7. What is the **generic name** for Biquin Durales (Canada)? _____

8. What is the **brand name** for esmolol? _____

9. What is the **generic name** for Xylocaine (United States) and Xylocard (Canada)? _____

10. What is the **brand name** for propranolol? _____

11. What is the **generic name** for Mexitil (United States)? _____

12. What is a **brand name** for amiodarone? _____

13. What is the **generic name** for Ethmozine (United States)? _____

14. What is the **generic name** for Betapace (United States) and Rylosol (Canada)? _____

15. What is the **generic name** for Isoptin? _____

MATCHING

Patient education is an essential component of therapeutics. Select the **best** warning label to apply to the prescription vial given to patients taking the drugs listed.

1. _____ quinidine SO_4 A. DILUTE ORAL CONCENTRATE

2. _____ disopyramide CR   B. AVOID PROLONGED EXPOSURE TO SUNLIGHT

3. _____ procainamide   C. SWALLOW WHOLE; DON'T CHEW

4. _____ propranolol 80 mg/mL   D. TAKE ON AN EMPTY STOMACH

5. _____ amiodarone   E. AVOID GRAPEFRUIT JUICE

MATCHING

Match each drug to its pharmacological classification.

1. _____ amiodarone   A. sodium channel blockade

2. _____ acebutolol   B. Ca^{2+} channel blockade

3. _____ lisinopril   C. K^+ channel blockade

4. _____ disopyramide   D. beta blocker

5. _____ verapamil   E. ACE inhibitor

TRUE OR FALSE

1. _____ Class I antiarrhythmic agents can produce local anesthesia.

2. _____ Antiarrhythmic drugs are categorized into classes I, II, III, IV, and V.

3. _____ Calcium channel blockers are the only class of drugs indicated for the primary management of ventricular arrhythmias.

4. _____ Class II antiarrhythmics (beta blockers) are contraindicated in patients with asthma, diabetes, and heart failure.

5. _____ Quinidine is the active ingredient in cinchona bark.

The following hard copies are brought to your pharmacy for filling. Identify the prescription error(s). (You already have the patient's full address on file.)

```
┌─────────────────────────────────────────────┐
│         Anh Dang Tu, MD        Date _____    │
│           1145 Broadway                       │
│           Anytown, USA                        │
│                                               │
│  Pt. Name _____ Lili Ng _____   │
│  Address _____    │
│  ℞   quinine SO4 300mg    #30                 │
│       1 tab TID for arrhythmia                │
│                                               │
│                                               │
│  Refills _____                               │
│                                               │
│  _____       AD Tu                 │
│  Substitution permitted    Dispense as written│
└─────────────────────────────────────────────┘
```

1. Spot the error in the following prescription:

   _____

   A. Quantity missing
   B. Directions incomplete
   C. Strength missing
   D. Strength incorrect
   E. Drug name incorrect

```
┌─────────────────────────────────────────────┐
│         Anh Dang Tu, MD        Date _____    │
│           1145 Broadway                       │
│           Anytown, USA                        │
│                                               │
│  Pt. Name _____ Sheila Alvater _____   │
│  Address _____    │
│  ℞   disopyramide CR   #30                    │
│       1 tab BID                               │
│                                               │
│                                               │
│  Refills _____                               │
│                                               │
│  _____       AD Tu                 │
│  Substitution permitted    Dispense as written│
└─────────────────────────────────────────────┘
```

2. Spot the error in the following prescription:

   _____

   A. Quantity missing
   B. Directions incomplete
   C. Strength missing
   D. Strength incorrect
   E. Dosage form incorrect

3. Give six pairs of drug names that have look-alike or sound-alike issues with drugs used to treat arrhythmias.

DRUG NAME	LOOK-ALIKE OR SOUND-ALIKE DRUG

RESEARCH ACTIVITY

1. Dan Cowan calls to renew his antiarrhythmic drug. He does not remember the name.

   Review his patient profile and then make a list of the medications that are used in the treatment of arrhythmia. Develop a list of questions you might ask to identify the drug he is requesting.

Last name: Cowan

First name: Dan

Gender: M

Address: 1906 E Denny Wy

City: Anytown

DOB: 02-13-46

Allergies: penicillin

Comment: $8/12 copay

Disc.:

Phone: 206-322-6789

Insurance: PC

Plan: 05

Group#: 12345678

ID#: 526458904

Copay: $8.00*

Cardholder: Cowan

Dan

Exp. date:

DATE	RX#	DRUG AND STRENGTH	SIG	QTY	MD	RF
1-2-08	72345	furosemide 40 mg	1 QD	100	Johnson	2
1-2-08	72346	K-Dur 20 mEq	1 BID	120	Johnson	3
2-2-08	81956	Niaspan 750 mg	1 BID	100	Johnson	
2-9-08	79278	ASA gr 5	1 QD	100	Johnson	1
2-9-08	79279	Monopril 10 mg	1 QD	30	Johnson	2
3-1-08	79279	Monopril 10 mg	1 QD	60	Johnson	1
4-25-08	84639	Lescol 40 mg	1 QD	30	Johnson	1
5-2-08	102344	Betapace 160 mg	1 BID	25	Johnson	4
5-2-08	96346	Ticlid 250 mg	1 BID	60	Johnson	1
5-23-08	100013	Lipitor 10 mg	1 qd	60	Johnson	
6-4-08	105278	Norpace CR 100 mg	1 BID	60	Johnson	
7-1-08	110129	amiodarone 200 mg	1 q12h	60	Johnson	

ANTIPARKINSON DRUG	DRUG IDENTIFICATION QUESTIONS
	1.
	2.
	3.

Treatment of Gastroesophageal Reflux Disease, Laryngopharyngeal Reflux, and Peptic Ulcer Disease

26

TERMS AND DEFINITIONS

Match each term with the correct definition below. Some terms may not be used.

A. Duodenal ulcer

B. Endoscopy

C. Gastroesophageal reflux disease (GERD)

D. Hiatal hernia

E. Laryngopharyngeal reflux (LPR)

F. Lower esophageal sphincter (LES)

G. Peristalsis

H. Peptic ulcer disease (PUD)

I. Reflux

J. Ulcer

K. Upper esophageal sphincter (UES)

L. Gastric ulcer

1. _____ is a motility disorder associated with impaired peristalsis.

2. The condition in which the lower esophageal sphincter shifts above the diaphragm is _____.

3. _____ is a forceful wave of contractions in the esophagus that moves food and liquids from the mouth to the stomach.

4. _____ is a test that uses a small video camera to look for ulcers inside of the stomach and small intestine.

5. Backflow or _____ of gastric contents into the esophagus or laryngopharyngeal region is responsible for symptoms of PUD and GERD.

6. _____ is a term that is used to describe ulcers that are located in either the duodenum or stomach.

7. The _____ separates the esophagus and the stomach.

8. An ulcer that is located in the upper portion of the small intestine or duodenum is called a(n) _____.

9. The _____ separates the pharynx and esophagus.

10. A(n) _____ is an open would or sore.

11. _____ is a condition in which gastric contents reflux into the larynx and pharynx.

12. A(n) _____ is an ulcer that is located in the stomach.

MULTIPLE CHOICE

1. Gastroesophageal reflux disease (GERD) is a motility disorder that results from the backflow

   of gastric contents into the _____.
   A. small intestine
   B. esophagus
   C. larynx
   D. pharynx

2. If left untreated, GERD may increase the risk for

   development of _____.
   A. stomach cancer
   B. asthma
   C. hemorrhage
   D. all of the above

3. All of the following may be used in the treatment of

   peptic ulcer disease *except* _____.
   A. cimetidine
   B. aluminum hydroxide gel
   C. sucralfate
   D. methylprednisolone
   E. lansoprazole

4. A patient taking an antacid preparation develops constipation. What combination of ingredients in antacids is likely to cause this side effect?

   _____
   A. magnesium hydroxide gel plus simethicone
   B. magaldrate plus simethicone
   C. aluminum hydroxide plus calcium carbonate
   D. aluminum hydroxide plus magnesium hydroxide gel

5. Which food and beverages do *not* aggravate GERD?

   _____
   A. fried food
   B. alcohol
   C. apple juice
   D. milk
   E. citrus fruits and tomato-based foods

6. Which treatment for GERD requires a prescription?

   _____
   A. Tagamet
   B. Axid
   C. Pepcid
   D. Nexium

7. The number one cause of peptic ulcer disease is

   _____.
   A. *H. pylori* infection
   B. stress
   C. drug therapy
   D. spicy foods

8. Ulcer formation is a possible adverse reaction of all

   of the following drugs *except* _____.
   A. aspirin
   B. lansoprazole
   C. NSAIDs
   D. prednisone

9. Select the drug that is administered to prevent the formation of ulcers in people who take NSAIDs.

   _____
   A. cimetidine
   B. sucralfate
   C. esomeprazole
   D. misoprostol

10. Which drug promotes healing of ulcers and acts like

    a "Band-Aid?" _____
    A. cimetidine
    B. sucralfate
    C. esomeprazole
    D. misoprostol

FILL IN THE BLANK: DRUG NAMES

1. What is the **brand name** for famotidine? _____

2. What is the **generic name** for Tagamet (United States)? _____

3. What is a **brand name** for nizatidine? _____

4. What is the **generic name** for Nexium? _____

5. What is the **generic name** for Prevacid? _____

6. What is the **generic name** for Prilosec (United States) and Losec (Canada)? _____

7. What is the **brand name** for misoprostol plus diclofenac? _____

8. What is the **generic name** for Protonix (United States) and Pantoloc (Canada)? _____

9. What is the **generic name** for Carafate (United States) and Sulcrate (Canada)? _____

10. What is the **generic name** for Aciphex (United States) and Pariet (Canada)? _____

11. What is the **generic name** for Prevpac (United States) and HP PAC (Canada)? _____

12. What is the **generic name** for Reglan (United States)? _____

13. What is the **generic name** for Cytotec (United States)? _____

MATCHING

Patient education is an essential component of therapeutics. Select the **best** warning label to apply to the prescription vial given to patients taking the drugs listed.

1. _____ misoprostol 100 microgram

2. _____ Prevacid 30 mg

3. _____ Pepcid 40 mg/5 ml

4. _____ metoclopramide 10 mg

5. _____ cimetidine 300 mg

A. SWALLOW WHOLE; DO NOT CRUSH OR CHEW

B. AVOID ALCOHOL

C. SHAKE WELL AND DISCARD AFTER 30 DAYS

D. MAY CAUSE DROWSINESS

E. AVOID PREGNANCY

TRUE OR FALSE

1. _____ Gastric ulcers are located in the small intestine.

2. _____ Reflux esophagitis is the name given to gastric ulcers.

3. _____ Misoprostol is given to prevent ulcers associated with the administration of NSAIDs.

4. _____ The main use of antacids is to provide a protective coating to the stomach lining.

5. _____ Stress and spicy foods can cause ulcers.

6. _____ A common ending for H$_2$ blockers is *-tidine*.

7. _____ Proton pump inhibitors have the common ending *-prazole*.

CRITICAL THINKING

The following hard copies are brought to your pharmacy for filling. Identify the prescription error(s). (You already have the patient's full address on file.)

Anh Dang Tu, MD   Date _____
1145 Broadway
Anytown, USA

Pt. Name _____ Jon Nguyen _____
Address _____

℞   nizatidine 300mg caps once daily at bedtime

Refills _____
_____ AD Tu _____
Substitution permitted   Dispense as written

1. Spot the error in the following prescription:

   _____

   A. Quantity missing
   B. Directions incomplete
   C. Strength missing
   D. Strength incorrect
   E. Dosage form incorrect

Anh Dang Tu, MD   Date _____
1145 Broadway
Anytown, USA

Pt. Name _____ Lili Ng _____
Address _____

℞   omeprazole 20mg   #30
    1/2 cap QD

Refills _____
_____ AD Tu _____
Substitution permitted   Dispense as written

2. Spot the error in the following prescription:

   _____

   A. Quantity missing
   B. Directions incorrect
   C. Strength missing
   D. Strength incorrect
   E. Dosage form incorrect

Anh Dang Tu, MD   Date _____
1145 Broadway
Anytown, USA

Pt. Name _____ Sean Price _____
Address _____

℞   Aciphex   #30
    i QD

Refills _____
_____ AD Tu _____
Substitution permitted   Dispense as written

3. Spot the error in the following prescription:

   _____

   A. Quantity missing
   B. Directions incomplete
   C. Strength missing
   D. Strength incorrect
   E. Dosage form incorrect

4. Give six pairs of drug names that have look-alike or sound-alike issues with drugs used to treat GERD, LPR, and PUD.

DRUG NAME	LOOK-ALIKE OR SOUND-ALIKE DRUG

5. Ms. Shorter is prescribed ranitidine 300 mg q HS. She is having difficulty swallowing the tablets and wants a liquid dosage form. Ranitidine is available 150 mg/tsp. How many milliliters must she take per dose? Please show your calculations.

_____

_____

_____

_____

_____

RESEARCH ACTIVITY

1. Lifestyle change is an important component of treatment and prevention of ulcers. What lifestyle changes are recommended? Access the National Library of Medicine's website (http://www.nlm.nih.gov/medlineplus/pepticulcer .html) to answer the question.

_____

_____

_____

_____

_____

27 Treatment of Irritable Bowel Syndrome, Ulcerative Colitis, and Crohn's Disease

TERMS AND DEFINITIONS

Match each term with the correct definition below. Some terms may not be used.

A. Antidiarrheals

B. Colonoscopy

C. Crohn disease

D. Fistula

E. Gastroenteritis

F. Inflammatory bowel disease (IBD)

G. Irritable bowel syndrome (IBS)

H. Laxatives

I. Toxic megacolon

J. Ulcer

K. Ulcerative colitis

L. Constipation

M. Diarrhea

1. _____ is an infection in the gastrointestinal tract that can cause postinfection irritable bowel syndrome.

2. Constipation is treated with _____, medicines that induce evacuation of the bowel.

3. A(n) _____ is a(n) _____ that tunnels from the site of origin to surrounding tissues.

4. _____ are used to reduce abnormally frequent passage of loose and watery stools.

5. _____ may produce constipation or diarrhea.

6. Inflammation of the colon that occurs with _____ causes ulcers and damage to the colon.

7. A person who has _____ has inflammation of the intestine, and _____ may produce inflammation anywhere along the GI tract.

8. _____ is a life-threatening condition characterized by a very inflated colon; abdominal distention; and sometimes fever, abdominal pain, or shock.

9. A(n) _____ is a diagnostic examination performed using an endoscope.

10. _____ is abnormally delayed or infrequent passage of dry, hardened feces.

11. Abnormally frequent passage of loose and watery stools is known as _____.

MULTIPLE CHOICE

1. Which of the following gastrointestinal conditions is *not* characterized by inflammation?

   _____
   A. irritable bowel disease
   B. ulcerative colitis
   C. irritable bowel syndrome
   D. Crohn disease

2. Select the **false** statement. _____
   A. Ulcerative colitis and Crohn disease are inflammatory bowel diseases.
   B. Irritable bowel syndrome may be associated with abnormally low levels of the neurotransmitter norepinephrine.
   C. In ulcerative colitis and Crohn disease, the body's immune system recognizes the bacteria that normally inhabit the GI tract as harmful invaders and releases anti–tumor necrosis factor (TNF).
   D. Ulcerative colitis produces inflammation in the upper layers of the lining of the small intestine and colon.
   E. Lifestyle modification can reduce symptoms of IBS, ulcerative colitis, and Crohn disease.

3. Which drug(s) may only be prescribed by physicians enrolled in a drug-specific prescribing program?

   _____
   A. sulfasalazine
   B. alosetron
   C. tegaserod
   D. fiber supplements
   E. loperamide

4. Which drug is *not* classified as an aminosalicylate?

   _____
   A. atropine
   B. mesalazine
   C. olsalazine
   D. balsalazide
   E. mesalamine

5. Which of the following lifestyle modifications can reduce symptoms of IBS, ulcerative colitis, and

   Crohn disease? _____
   A. stress management
   B. eating small meals
   C. avoiding alcohol
   D. avoiding caffeinated and carbonated beverages
   E. all of the above

6. Which statement about glucocorticosteroid use for the treatment of Crohn disease is **false**?

   _____
   A. Glucocorticosteroids decrease inflammation.
   B. Glucocorticosteroids increase inflammation.
   C. Glucocorticosteroids are immunosuppressants.
   D. Glucocorticosteroids reduce flare-ups.

7. Which drug does *not* induce remission of Crohn

   disease? _____
   A. azathioprine
   B. infliximab
   C. 6-mercaptopurine
   D. methotrexate
   E. olsalazine

FILL IN THE BLANK: DRUG NAMES

1. What is the *generic name* for Lotronex (United States.)? _____

2. What is the *brand name* for diphenoxylate plus atropine? _____

3. What is the *generic name* for Atreza (United States)? _____

4. What is the *generic name* for Bentyl (United States) and Bentylol (Canada)? _____

5. What is the *generic name* for Colazal (United States)? _____

6. What is the *brand name* for mesalamine (United States) and mesalazine (Canada)? _____

7. What is the **brand name** for olsalazine? _____

8. What is the **generic name** for Azulfadine (United States) and Salazopyrin (Canada)? _____

9. What is a **brand name** for 5-aminosalicylic acid (5-ASA)? _____

10. What is a **generic name** for Cortifoam? _____

11. What is a **generic name** for Winpred (Canada)? _____

12. What is the **generic name** for Decadron (United States) and Dexasone (Canada)? _____

13. What is the **brand name** for methylprednisolone? _____

14. What is the **generic name** for Imuran? _____

15. What is the **brand name** for 6-mercaptopurine? _____

16. What is a **generic name** for Trexall (United States)? _____

17. What is a **brand name** for infliximab? _____

MATCHING

Match each drug to its therapeutic classification.

1. _____ hydrocortisone enema   A. serotonin receptor antagonist

2. _____ alosetron 1 mg tab   B. immunosuppressant

3. _____ methotrexate 2.5 mg tab   C. serotonin receptor partial agonist

4. _____ infliximab 100 mg   D. imunomodulator

     E. corticosteroid

MATCHING

Match each drug to its therapeutic classification.

1. _____ olsalazine 250 mg cap   A. immunosuppressant

2. _____ loperamide 2 mg   B. anticholinergic

3. _____ Imuran 50 mg tab   C. corticosteroid

4. _____ dicyclomine 20 mg tab   D. antidiarrheal

5. _____ methylprednisolone 4 mg   E. aminosalicylate

TRUE OR FALSE

1. _____ Crohn disease only produces inflammation and damage in the colon.

2. _____ Infliximab is an immunomodulator.

3. _____ Inflammatory bowel disease (IBD) and irritable bowel syndrome (IBS) are the same condition.

4. _____ Irritable bowel syndrome may be associated with abnormally low levels of the neurotransmitter serotonin.

5. _____ Toxic megacolon is a life-threatening adverse effect of Alosetron.

6. _____ All commercially available aminosalicylates (5-ASA) are formulated as delayed-release products.

7. _____ Ulcerative colitis most commonly occurs between the ages of 30 and 50 years.

CRITICAL THINKING

The following hard copies are brought to your pharmacy for filling. Identify the prescription error(s). (You already have the patient's full address on file.)

| Anh Dang Tu, MD | Date _____ |
| 1145 Broadway |
| Anytown, USA |

Pt. Name _____ Wilma Russell _____

Address _____

R͟x Zelnorm   #30
      i tab BID

Refills _____

_____   _____ Tu _____
Substitution permitted   Dispense as written

1. Spot the error in the following prescription:

   _____

   A. Quantity missing
   B. Directions incomplete
   C. Strength missing
   D. Strength incorrect
   E. Dosage form incorrect

| Kathy Principi, MD | Date _____ |
| 1145 Broadway |
| Anytown, USA |

Pt. Name _____ Will Jones _____

Address _____

R͟x Pentasa #28
      Insert rectally as directed

Refills _____

____ Principi ____   _____
Substitution permitted   Dispense as written

2. Spot the error in the following prescription:

   _____

   A. Quantity missing
   B. Directions incomplete
   C. Refills missing
   D. Strength incorrect
   E. Dosage form missing

1. How is the function of the immune system linked to ulcerative colitis and Crohn disease? Access the National Digestive Diseases Information Clearing house's website (http://www.digestive.niddk.nih.gov) to answer the question.

_____

_____

_____

_____

_____

28 Treatment of Asthma and Chronic Obstructive Pulmonary Disease

TERMS AND DEFINITIONS

Match each term with the correct definition below. Some terms may not be used.

A. Allergic asthma

B. Asthma

C. Bronchodilators

D. Chronic obstructive pulmonary disease (COPD)

E. Forced expiratory volume

F. Nebulizer

G. Peak flow meter

H. Spacer

I. Spirometry

J. Metered-dose inhaler (MDI)

1. Two tests that measure volume of air are _____ and _____.

2. _____ is a progressive disease of the airways that produces gradual loss of pulmonary function.

3. _____ is typically defined as a chronic disease that affects the airways producing irritation, inflammation, and difficulty breathing; however, symptoms of _____ occur upon exposure to environmental allergens.

4. Whereas corticosteroids are used in the treatment of asthma to reduce inflammation and swelling of airways, _____ relax tightened airway muscles.

5. Devices that are used to improve the delivery of inhaled medicines are _____ and _____.

6. The _____ is a handheld device that is used to measure the volume of air exhaled and how fast the air is moved out.

7. _____ is a device used for delivering a dose of inhaled medication. A solution or powder is delivered as a mist and inhaled.

MULTIPLE CHOICE

1. Symptoms of asthma include all of the following

   except _____.
   A. coughing
   B. wheezing
   C. sneezing
   D. shortness of breath
   E. chest tightness

2. Asthma triggers include all of the following *except*

   _____.
   A. mild exercise
   B. cockroach droppings
   C. environmental and household pollutants
   D. tobacco smoke
   E. air pollution

3. Treatment of COPD involves the administration of

   _____.
   A. bronchodilators
   B. glucocorticosteroids
   C. antibiotics when infections are present
   D. oxygen
   E. all of the above

4. Which of the following drugs is *not* a "reliever" medicine prescribed for the treatment of acute

   symptoms of asthma? _____
   A. albuterol (or salbutamol)
   B. levalbuterol
   C. beclomethasone
   D. terbutaline
   E. ipratropium bromide

5. Which of the following classes of drugs is *not* a "controller" medicine, prescribed to prevent

   symptoms of asthma? _____
   A. long-acting β_2-agonists
   B. short-acting β_2-agonists
   C. inhaled corticosteroids
   D. leukotriene modifiers
   E. mast cell stabilizers

6. Which of the following drugs is *not* inhaled orally?

   _____
   A. Flovent
   B. Pulmicort
   C. Azmacort
   D. Qvar
   E. Rhinocort

7. Select the **false** statement. _____
   A. Leukotriene modifiers are administered to patients with mild asthma to reduce inflammation.
   B. Leukotriene modifiers inhibit the release of proinflammatory substances.
   C. The packet of montelukast granules may be opened and premixed hours in advance for convenience.
   D. Montelukast granules may be mixed in food.

FILL IN THE BLANK: DRUG NAMES

1. What is a *generic name* for Ventolin? _____

2. What is the *generic name* for Xopenex (United States)? _____

3. What is the *generic name* for Alupent (United States)? _____

4. What is the *generic name* for Maxair (United States)? _____

5. What is the *brand name* for albuterol plus ipratropium bromide? _____

6. What is the *brand name* for fenoterol hydrobromide plus ipratropium bromide? _____

7. What is the *generic name* for Foradil? _____

8. What is the *generic name* for Serevent Diskus? _____

9. What is the *generic name* for Qvar? _____

10. What is the **brand name** for budesonide? _____

11. What is the **brand name** for fluticasone? _____

12. What is the **generic name** for Azmacort (United States)? _____

13. What is the **brand name** for formoterol plus budesonide? _____

14. What is the **generic name** for Singulair? _____

15. What is the **generic name** for Accolate? _____

16. What is the **generic name** for Zyflo CR (United States)? _____

17. What is a **brand name** for theophylline? _____

18. What is a **brand name** for omalizumab? _____

MATCHING

Patient education is an essential component of therapeutics. Select the **best** warning label to apply to the prescription vial given to patients taking the drugs listed.

1. _____ omalizumab

2. _____ beclomethasone inh

3. _____ Accolate 20 mg tab

4. _____ theophylline 200 mg SR

A. TAKE ON AN EMPTY STOMACH

B. SWALLOW WHOLE; DON'T CRUSH OR CHEW

C. REFRIGERATE; DO NOT FREEZE

D. SHAKE WELL

MATCHING

Match each drug to its therapeutic classification.

1. _____ Pulmicort

2. _____ Advair

3. _____ Ventolin inhaler

4. _____ salmeterol

5. _____ zafirlukast 10 mg tab

A. short-acting β_2-adrenergic agonists

B. long-acting β_2-adrenergic agonists

C. inhaled corticosteroids

D. long-acting β_2-adrenergic agonist plus corticosteroid

E. leukotriene modifiers

TRUE OR FALSE

1. _____ An MDI canister will float to the top of a jar of water when the contents are full.

2. _____ Long-acting β_2-adrenergic agonists (e.g., salmeterol) have been associated with an increased risk of severe asthma exacerbations and asthma-related death.

3. _____ A common ending for leukotriene modifiers is *-lukast*.

4. _____ A common ending for xanthine derivatives is *-phylline*.

5. _____ A common ending for monoclonal antibody drugs is *-mab*.

6. _____ Asthma symptoms cannot be managed with lifestyle modification only.

7. _____ Chronic obstructive pulmonary disease (COPD) is an acute disease.

8. _____ Exposure to second-hand smoke and air pollution are risk factors for developing asthma.

9. _____ The use of orally inhaled corticosteroids may cause thrush (a "yeast" infection).

CRITICAL THINKING

The following hard copies are brought to your pharmacy for filling. Identify the prescription error(s). (You already have the patient's full address on file.)

```
┌─────────────────────────────────────────┐
│         Anh Dang Tu, MD      Date _____ │
│         1145 Broadway                    │
│         Anytown, USA                     │
│                                          │
│ Pt. Name _____ Wilbur Wolf _____ │
│ Address _____ │
│ ℞   Serevent Diskus   #1                 │
│       1-2 inhalations every 4-6 hours    │
│                                          │
│                                          │
│ Refills _____                           │
│                              Tu          │
│ _____     _____    │
│ Substitution permitted   Dispense as written │
└─────────────────────────────────────────┘
```

1. Spot the error in the following prescription:

   _____

   A. Quantity missing
   B. Directions incorrect
   C. Strength missing
   D. Strength incorrect
   E. Dosage form missing

```
┌─────────────────────────────────────────┐
│         Kathy Principi, MD   Date _____ │
│         1145 Broadway                    │
│         Anytown, USA                     │
│                                          │
│ Pt. Name _____ Will Jones _____ │
│ Address _____ │
│ ℞   Singular chewable tablets  #30       │
│       Chew and swallow 1 tablet daily    │
│                                          │
│                                          │
│ Refills _____                           │
│       Principi                           │
│ _____     _____    │
│ Substitution permitted   Dispense as written │
└─────────────────────────────────────────┘
```

2. Spot the error in the following prescription:

   _____

   A. Quantity missing
   B. Directions incomplete
   C. Strength missing
   D. Strength incorrect
   E. Dosage form missing

RESEARCH ACTIVITY

Access the National Institute of Environmental Health Sciences' website (http://www.niehs.nih.gov) and the National Heart, Lung, and Blood Institute's website (http://www.nhlbi.nih.gov/health/dci/Diseases/Asthma/) to answer the following questions.

1. The prevalence of asthma is increasing in large urban cities. What might account for this trend?

_____

_____

_____

_____

_____

2. Explain the following analogy. "The peak flow meter is to asthma management as the blood glucose monitor is to diabetes management."

_____

_____

_____

_____

_____

29 Treatment of Allergies

TERMS AND DEFINITIONS

Match each term with the correct definition below. Some terms may not be used.

A. Allergen

B. Allergic rhinitis

C. Allergy

D. Anaphylaxis

E. Angioedema

F. Mast cells

G. Wheal

H. Allergic conjunctivitis

I. Histamine

J. Immunoglobulin E

K. Leukotriene

L. Urticaria

1. A(n) _____ is a hypersensitivity reaction by the immune system upon exposure to an

   _____.

2. Persons who have _____ experience seasonal or perennial nasal swelling and a runny nose.

3. _____ is a life-threatening allergic reaction.

4. The medical term for a raised blisterlike area on the skin caused by allergic reaction is _____.

5. An allergic response begins with the release of _____, granule-containing cells found in tissue.

6. _____ may be life threatening if swelling involves the mucous membranes and the viscera.

7. A(n) _____ is an organic nitrogen compound involved in local immune responses as well as regulating physiological function in the gut and acting as a neurotransmitter.

8. _____ is known as hives.

9. _____ is a proinflammatory mediator released as part of the allergic, inflammatory response.

10. _____ is known as inflammation of the tissue lining the eyelids caused by the reaction to an allergy-causing substance.

11. _____ is an antibody that *is* associated with allergies.

MULTIPLE CHOICE

1. Symptoms of seasonal allergic rhinitis (SAR) include all of the following *except* _____.
   A. runny nose
   B. rash
   C. itching nose
   D. stuffy nose

2. Which of the following is *not* a mediator of the allergic response? _____
   A. CD4$^+$ T-lymphocytes
   B. CD81
   C. interleukin-4 (IL-4)
   D. interleukin-6 (IL-6)
   E. immunoglobulin E (IgE)

3. Which of the following is a common allergen? _____
   A. Cat dander
   B. Dust
   C. Mold
   D. Pollen
   E. All of the above

4. Pharmacy technicians are at risk for developing latex allergy. Symptoms of latex allergy include all of the following *except* _____.
   A. sneezing
   B. itchy eyes
   C. scratchy throat
   D. hives
   E. blurred vision

5. Drugs used to treat allergic symptoms include all of the following *except* _____.
   A. fexofenadine
   B. Rhinocort AQ
   C. cromolyn
   D. pseudoephedrine
   E. Nasacort

6. Which of the following antihistamines requires a prescription in the United States? _____
   A. diphenhydramine
   B. desloratadine
   C. loratadine
   D. cetirizine
   E. clemastine

7. Steps to protect oneself from latex exposure and allergy in the workplace include _____.
   A. select nonlatex gloves when possible
   B. use powder-free latex gloves with reduced protein content
   C. avoid oil-based hand creams and lotions when wearing latex gloves
   D. wash hands with a mild soap and dry thoroughly after removing latex gloves
   E. all of the above

FILL IN THE BLANK: DRUG NAMES

1. What are **brand names** for desloratadine? _____

2. What is the **generic name** for Allegra? _____

3. What is the **brand name** for beclomethasone AQ? _____

4. What is the **generic name** for Rhinocort Aqua? _____

5. What are **brand names** for flunisolide? _____

6. What is the **generic name** Flonase? _____

7. What is the **brand name** for fluticasone furoate? _____

8. What is the *generic name* for Nasacort AQ? _____

9. What is the *brand name* for cromolyn sodium? _____

MATCHING

Patient education is an essential component of therapeutics. Select the **best** warning label to apply to the prescription vial given to patients taking the drugs listed.

1. _____ diphenhydramine 50 mg   A. AVOID GRAPEFRUIT JUICE

2. _____ Allegra 24 hour   B. SWALLOW WHOLE; DON'T CRUSH OR CHEW

3. _____ loratadine disintegrating tabs   C. PROTECT FROM MOISTURE

4. _____ fexofenadine   D. SHAKE WELL

5. _____ Flonase   E. MAY CAUSE DROWSINESS

MATCHING

Match each drug to its therapeutic classification.

1. _____ cromolyn sodium   A. antihistamine

2. _____ Rhinocort Aqua   B. mast cell stabilizer

3. _____ desloratadine 5 mg   C. inhaled corticosteroids

TRUE OR FALSE

1. _____ The immune system treats the allergen as an invader and produces antibodies to the substance.

2. _____ The production of allergen-specific IgE antibodies and T-cell responses directed against allergens develop after age 7 years.

3. _____ The six classes of antihistamines are ethylenediamines, ethanolamines, alkylamines, piperazines, phenothiazines, and cimetidine.

4. _____ Pharmacy technicians are at risk for developing latex allergy.

5. _____ Sedation is the most common side effect of loratadine.

6. _____ The use of intranasal corticosteroids may cause nosebleeds and a sore throat.

7. _____ Diphenhydramine is used to treat allergy symptoms and insomnia.

CRITICAL THINKING

The following hard copies are brought to your pharmacy for filling. Identify the prescription error(s). (You already have the patient's full address on file.)

Anh Dang Tu, MD Date _____ 1145 Broadway Anytown, USA Pt. Name _____ Wilbur Wolf _____ Address _____ ℞ *Rhinocort Aqua inhaler #1* *1-2 spray each nostril 2-3 times a day* Refills _____ _____ _____ *Tu* _____ Substitution permitted Dispense as written	1. Spot the error in the following prescription: _____ A. Quantity missing B. Directions incorrect C. Strength missing D. Strength incorrect E. Dosage form missing

Kathy Principi, MD Date _____ 1145 Broadway Anytown, USA Pt. Name _____ Will Jones _____ Address _____ ℞ *desloratadine syrup 0.5mg/ml* *1-2 teaspoonfuls daily* Refills _____ *Principi* _____ _____ Substitution permitted Dispense as written	2. Spot the error in the following prescription: _____ A. Quantity missing B. Directions incomplete C. Strength missing D. Strength incorrect E. Dosage form missing

RESEARCH ACTIVITY

1. What is the link between allergies and air pollution? Access the National Institute of Allergy and Infectious Disease's website (http://www.niaid.nih.gov) and other websites to answer the question.

_____

_____

_____

_____

_____

30 Treatment of Prostate Disease and Erectile Dysfunction

TERMS AND DEFINITIONS

Match each term with the correct definition below. Some terms may not be used.

A. Benign prostatic hyperplasia (BPH)

B. Digital rectal examination (DRE)

C. Erectile dysfunction (ED)

D. Urinary frequency

E. Hyperplasia

F. Incontinence

G. Prostate gland

H. Prostate-specific antigen (PSA)

I. Prostatitis

J. Prostate-specific antigen (PSA) test

K. Urinalysis

L. Urinary urgency

M. alpha blockers

N. α-Reductase inhibitor

O. Ejaculation

P. Phosphodiesterase type 5 inhibitor (PDE5)

Q. Semen

R. Tumor

1. _____ is defined as the persistent inability to achieve or maintain an erection sufficient for satisfactory sexual intercourse.

2. The _____ and _____ are screening exams for prostate disease (cancer and BPH).

3. _____ is a protein that is elevated in men who have prostate cancer, infection, or inflammation of the prostate gland and BPH.

4. _____ is inflammation of the _____ gland.

5. BPH and infections may produce _____, the need to urinate more often than normal.

6. _____ is a microscopic and chemical examination of a fresh urine sample that is used to screen for infection.

7. _____ is a loss of bladder or bowel control.

8. One symptom of BPH is _____, the feeling of needing to urinate immediately.

9. _____ is a noncancerous growth of cells in the prostate gland.

10. The medical term for an abnormal increase in the number of cells in an organ or tissue is _____.

11. _____ is a drug that shrinks the prostate gland; it is used to treat BPH.

12. _____ is the release of semen from the penis during orgasm.

13. A _____ is an abnormal mass of tissue that results from excessive cell division.

14. _____ is the fluid containing sperm and secretions from glands of the male reproductive tract.

15. _____ are drugs used in the treatment of benign prostatic hyperplasia to relax muscles in the prostate and increase urine flow.

16. _____ is a drug used to relax smooth muscle and blood vessels that supply the corpus cavernosum and control penile engorgement.

MULTIPLE CHOICE

1. Which of the following is *not* a benefit of α_1-adrenergic antagonists for the treatment of BPH? _____
   A. Relaxation of the prostate gland
   B. Increase of urethral resistance
   C. Improvement in flow of urine
   D. Relaxation of smooth muscle of the bladder

2. _____, an antiandrogen, is prescribed for benign prostatic hyperplasia and male pattern baldness.
   A. Finasteride
   B. Dutasteride
   C. Progesterone
   D. Testosterone

3. Which of the following drugs prescribed for the treatment of BPH is *not* an α_1. receptor blocking drug? _____
   A. alfuzosin
   B. Hytrin
   C. tamsulosin
   D. Proscar

4. The therapeutic effects of 5α-reductase inhibitors may take _____ months to be achieved.
   A. 1 to 2
   B. 3 to 6
   C. 6 to 12
   D. 12 to 18

5. The pharmacist should advise males taking finasteride and dutasteride _____.
   A. to use barrier contraceptives such as condoms
   B. that pregnant women and women of childbearing age should avoid contact with broken or crushed tablets
   C. may decrease desire for sex
   D. may cause erectile dysfunction
   E. all of the above

6. Which factor is *not* a cause of erectile dysfunction?

_____

A. lifestyle
B. heredity
C. psychological
D. physical
E. neurologic

7. Select the **false** statement about drugs used for the treatment of erectile dysfunction. _____

A. Sildenafil, tadalafil, and vardenafil are classified as phosphodiesterase type 5 (PDE5) inhibitors.
B. Cialis constricts smooth muscle and decreases the blood supply to the blood vessels that control penile engorgement.
C. Sildenafil, tadalafil, and vardenafil are contraindicated in patients taking nitroglycerin.
D. Alprostadil must be inserted into the urethra or by intracavernosal injection.

FILL IN THE BLANK: DRUG NAMES

1. What is the *generic name* for Uroxatral (United States) and Xatral (Canada)? _____

2. What is the *brand name* for doxazosin? _____

3. What is the *generic name* for Hytrin? _____

4. What is the *generic name* for Flomax? _____

5. What is the *brand name* for dutasteride? _____

6. What is the *generic name* for Proscar? _____

7. What are *brand names* for sildenafil? _____

8. What is the *generic name* for Cialis? _____

9. What is the *generic name* for Levitra? _____

10. What are *brand names* for alprostadil? _____

MATCHING

Patient education is an essential component of therapeutics. Select the **best** warning label to apply to the prescription vial given to patients taking the drugs listed.

1. _____ tamsulosin

2. _____ Proscar

3. _____ Cialis

4. _____ alprostadil inserts

A. AVOID GRAPEFRUIT JUICE

B. SWALLOW WHOLE; DON'T CRUSH OR CHEW

C. AVOID CONTACT WITH PREGNANT WOMEN

D. REFRIGERATE; DON'T FREEZE

MATCHING

Match each drug to its therapeutic classification.

1. _____ dutasteride
2. _____ tadalafil
3. _____ terazosin
4. _____ alprostadil

A. α_1-adrenergic antagonists

B. 5α-reductase inhibitors

C. phosphodiesterase-type inhibitors

D. prostaglandins

TRUE OR FALSE

1. _____ Saw palmetto is an herbal remedy for BPH.

2. _____ Saw palmetto may decrease the effect(s) of finasteride.

3. _____ Aggressive treatment for BPH is recommended when patients are asymptomatic or symptoms do not produce much discomfort.

4. _____ A common ending for 5α-reductase inhibitors is *-steride*.

5. _____ A common ending for phosphodiesterase-type inhibitors is *-afil*.

6. _____ A common ending for α_1-adrenergic antagonists is *-zosin*.

7. _____ By age 55 years, approximately 15% to 25% of men have erectile dysfunction.

CRITICAL THINKING

The following hard copies are brought to your pharmacy for filling. Identify the prescription error(s). (You already have the patient's full address on file.)

Anh Dang Tu, MD
1145 Broadway
Anytown, USA   Date _____
 	
Pt. Name _____ Wilbur Wolf _____
Address _____
℞ Flomax 0.4mg tablet   #30
     1 tablet daily
 	
Refills _____
 	
_____   ___ *Tu* ___
Substitution permitted   Dispense as written
	1. Spot the error in the following prescription:
	
	   _____
	
	   A. Quantity missing
	   B. Directions incomplete
	   C. Strength missing
	   D. Strength incorrect
	   E. Dosage form incorrect

```
┌──────────────────────────────────────┐
│           Kathy Principi, MD    Date _____   │
│              1145 Broadway            │
│              Anytown, USA             │
│                                       │
│  Pt. Name _____Will Jones_____   │
│  Address _____  │
│  ℞   Levitra 10mg  #10                │
│        1 tablet up to 60 minutes prior to sexual intercourse.│
│        May take up to 3 doses per day if desired│
│                                       │
│  Refills _____                       │
│  _____Principi_____   _____ │
│  Substitution permitted   Dispense as written│
└──────────────────────────────────────┘
```

2. Spot the error in the following prescription:

   _____

   A. Quantity missing
   B. Directions incorrect
   C. Strength missing
   D. Strength incorrect
   E. Dosage form missing

RESEARCH ACTIVITY

1. Write a paragraph describing lifestyle factors that contribute to erectile dysfunction. What changes should be made to improve treatment success? Access the National Library of Medicine's website (http://www.nlm.nih.gov/medlineplus/erectiledysfunction.html) to answer the question.

   _____

   _____

   _____

   _____

   _____

31 Treatment of Fluid and Electrolyte Disorders

TERMS AND DEFINITIONS

Match each term with the correct definition below. Some terms may not be used.

A. Chloride

B. Hyperchloremia

C. Hypochloremia

D. Hypernatremia

E. Hyperkalemia

F. Hypertonic

G. Hypokalemia

H. Hyponatremia

I. Hypotonic

J. Isotonic fluids

K. Magnesium

L. Potassium

M. Sodium

N. Crystalloids

O. Anion

P. Bicarbonate

Q. Cation

R. Osmolarity

S. Dehydration

T. Edema

U. Electrolytes

V. Extracellular fluid

W. Homeostasis

X. Intracellular fluid

Y. Ions

Z. Milliequivalent

AA. Osmolarity

BB. Colloids

CC. Hypomagnesemia

DD. Hypermagnesemia

EE. Hypophosphatemia

1. A deficient level of chloride in the blood is called _____; excess levels are called

   _____.

2. A deficient level of potassium in the blood is called _____; excess levels are called

   _____.

3. A deficient level of sodium in the blood is called _____; excess levels are called

   _____.

4. Positively charged ions include _____, _____, and _____.

5. IV solutions called _____ contain electrolytes in concentrations resembling those of plasma.

6. _____ fluids have the same osmolarity as serum, _____ fluids have less osmolarity

   than serum, and _____ fluids have a higher osmolarity than serum.

7. _____ are units used to measure the number of ionic charges or electrovalent bonds (electrolytes)
   in a solution.

8. Charged particles are known as _____.

9. _____ is the condition in which the serum phosphate level is defined as mild (2–2.5 mg/dL or
   0.65–0.81 mmol/L), moderate (1–2 mg/dL or 0.32–0.65 mmol/L), or severe (<1 mg/dL or 0.32 mmol/L).

10. _____ is the osmotic pressure of a solution expressed as osmoles or millimoles per liter
    (mmol/L) of the solution.

11. _____ is the type of fluid that surrounds the cells and consists mainly of the plasma found in
    blood vessels.

12. _____ is known as a negatively charged particle.

13. _____ are proteins or other large molecules that remain suspended in the blood for a long period
    of time and are too large to cross membranes.

14. _____ is fluid inside the cells.

15. _____ is a condition in which the serum level of magnesium exceeds 2.5 mEq/L.

16. The presence of abnormally large amounts of fluid in the intercellular tissue spaces of the body is known as

    _____.

17. _____ is the constancy or balance that is maintained by the body despite constant changes.

18. A positively charged electrolyte is known as a(n) _____.

19. _____ are small, charged molecules essential for homeostasis that play an important role in body chemistry.

20. _____ is the term used to describe the condition that results from excessive loss of body water.

21. _____ is the condition in which the serum level of magnesium is below 1.5 mEq/L.

22. The substance used as a buffer to maintain the normal levels of acidity (pH) in blood and other fluids in the

    body is known as _____.

MULTIPLE CHOICE

1. Electrolyte imbalances are caused by

   _____.
   A. hormonal or endocrine disorders
   B. kidney disease
   C. dehydration
   D. inadequate diet, lack of dietary vitamins, and malabsorption
   E. all of the above

2. Intravenous solutions that are used to treat fluid and

   electrolyte disorders may be _____.
   A. isotonic
   B. hypotonic
   C. hypertonic
   D. all of the above
   E. none of the above

3. Select the **false** statement. _____
   A. A hypotonic solution has less osmolarity than serum.
   B. A colloid solution contains electrolytes in concentrations less than plasma.
   C. A hypertonic solution has higher osmolarity than serum.
   D. An isotonic solution has the same osmolarity as serum.

4. Select the **true** statement about diuretics.

   _____
   A. Thiazide diuretics may produce hyperkalemia.
   B. Diuretics are used to treat edema.
   C. Diuretics may produce hypernatremia.
   D. Diuretics may produce edema.

5. Select the **false** statement. _____
   A. Hyperkalemia may be caused by excessive use of salt substitutes.
   B. Hyperkalemia is a side effect of potassium-sparing diuretics.
   C. Hyperkalemia is a side effect of K-Lyte.
   D. Hyperkalemia is a serum potassium level below 3.5mEq/L.

FILL IN THE BLANK: DRUG NAMES

1. What is the *generic name* for K-Lyte? _____

2. What is the *generic name* for Bumex (United States) and Burinex (Canada)? _____

3. What is the *brand name* for furosemide? _____

4. What is the *generic name* for Demadex (United States)? _____

MATCHING

Patient education is an essential component of therapeutics. Select the **best** warning label to apply to the prescription vial given to patients taking the drugs listed.

1. _____ calcium carbonate 600 mg

2. _____ potassium chloride powder

3. _____ furosemide 20 mg

A. DILUTE WITH WATER OR JUICE

B. AVOID FERROUS SUPPLEMENTS WITHIN 1 to 2 HOURS OF DOSE

C. AVOID PROLONGED EXPOSURE TO SUNLIGHT

MATCHING

Match each drug to its therapeutic classification.

1. _____ K-Lyte

2. _____ dextrose 5% in sterile water

3. _____ bumetanide 1 mg

4. _____ 0.45% sodium chloride

5. _____ 0.9% sodium chloride

A. loop diuretics

B. potassium replacement

C. normal saline

D. hypotonic solution

E. isotonic solution

TRUE OR FALSE

1. _____ Electrolytes are essential to many body functions, such as nerve conduction, muscle contraction, and bone growth.

2. _____ Extracellular fluid consists mainly of the plasma found in the blood vessels and the interstitial fluid in the cells.

3. _____ Dehydration may be caused by excessive use of diuretics.

4. _____ Rapidly drinking an excessive amount of fluids may cause a life-threatening electrolyte disorder.

5. _____ Hyponatremia may be treated by taking salt tablets.

CRITICAL THINKING

The following hard copy is brought to your pharmacy for filling. Identify the prescription error(s). (You already have the patient's full address on file.)

```
┌─────────────────────────────────────────┐
│      Marc Cordova, MD       Date _____ │
│         1145 Broadway                    │
│         Anytown, USA                     │
│                                          │
│ Pt. Name _____ Bill Carey _____ │
│ Address _____ │
│ Rx   bumetanide 10mg tab   #30           │
│       1 tablet daily                     │
│                                          │
│                                          │
│ Refills _____                          │
│   Cordova                                │
│ _____       _____   │
│ Substitution permitted   Dispense as written │
└─────────────────────────────────────────┘
```

1. Spot the error in the following prescription:

   _____

   A. Quantity missing
   B. Directions incomplete
   C. Strength missing
   D. Strength incorrect
   E. Dosage form missing

RESEARCH ACTIVITY

1. Prolonged diarrhea may cause dehydration and electrolyte imbalance. What are nonpharmacological methods to treat diarrhea and replenish electrolytes? Access the Merck Manual Online's website (http://www.merck.com/mmpe/index/ind_da.html) to answer the following question.

   _____

   _____

   _____

   _____

   _____

32 Treatment of Thyroid Disorders

TERMS AND DEFINITIONS

Match each term with the correct definition below. Some terms may not be used.

A. Antithyroid drugs

B. Graves disease

C. Hashimoto disease

D. Hypothyroidism

E. Hyperthyroidism

F. Radioactive iodine uptake (RAIU)

G. Thyroid antibody test

H. Thyroid-releasing factor (TRF)

I. Thyroid-stimulating hormone (TSH)

J. Tetraiodothyronine (T_4)

K. Triiodothyronine (T_3)

L. Thyroid-stimulating hormone (TSH) test

M. Tetraiodothyronine (T_4) test

1. A hormone released by the pituitary gland that stimulates the thyroid gland to produce and release thyroid

   hormones is _____.

2. _____ is a hormone released by the hypothalamus that stimulates the pituitary gland to release
   thyroid stimulating hormone.

3. Hormones released by the thyroid gland are _____ and _____.

4. _____, a condition in which there is an excessive production of thyroid hormones, is also called

   _____.

5. _____, a condition in which there is an insufficient production of thyroid hormones, is also called

   _____.

6. _____ is a diagnostic test to measure the level of thyroid-stimulating hormone in the blood.

7. The _____ is a diagnostic test used to measure levels of thyroid antibodies that are diagnostic for autoimmune thyroid disease.

8. The _____ measures "free" circulating thyroid hormone.

9. The _____ is a test that uses radioactive iodine to screen for thyroid disease.

10. A group of drugs administered to treat hyperthyroidism are called _____.

MULTIPLE CHOICE

1. All of the following may be used in the treatment of

    hyperthyroidism *except* _____.
    A. methimazole
    B. levothyroxine
    C. propylthiouracil
    D. radioactive iodine

2. What warning label should be applied to a prescription

    for methimazole 5 mg tab? _____
    A. AVOID PREGNANCY
    B. AVOID FERROUS PRODUCTS OR MULTIPLE VITAMINS WITHIN 4 HOURS OF DOSE
    C. AVOID ALCOHOL
    D. SWALLOW WHOLE; DO NOT CRUSH OR CHEW
    E. AVOID PROLONGED EXPOSURE TO SUNLIGHT

3. What warning label should be applied to a prescription

    for levothyroxine 0.05 mg tab? _____
    A. AVOID PREGNANCY
    B. AVOID FERROUS PRODUCTS OR MULTIPLE VITAMINS WITHIN 4 HOURS OF DOSE
    C. AVOID ALCOHOL
    D. SWALLOW WHOLE; DO NOT CRUSH OR CHEW
    E. AVOID PROLONGED EXPOSURE TO SUNLIGHT

4. Hormones secreted by the thyroid gland are

    _____.
    A. tetraiodothyronine (T_4)
    B. triiodothyronine (T_3)
    C. calcitonin
    D. all of the above

5. Select the **false** statement. _____
    A. When thyroid antibodies are present, autoimmune thyroid disease is diagnosed.
    B. Low-dose radioactive iodine (^{131}I) is administered to measure the amount of radioactivity take up by the thyroid gland.
    C. High-dose ^{131}I is administered to treat hyperthyroidism.
    D. Graves disease is an autoimmune disease that causes hypothyroidism.
    E. The full effects of ^{131}I therapy are achieved after 2 to 3 months in most people.

6. Select the **false** statement. _____
    A. It takes 2 to 4 months of therapy with propylthiouracil before maximum effects are achieved.
    B. Hashimoto disease is an autoimmune disorder that causes hyperthyroidism.
    C. Propylthiouracil (PTU) and methimazole block the synthesis of T_4 and T_3.
    D. Treatment with antithyroid drugs and radioactive iodine typically induces hypothyroidism.
    E. Synthetic T_4, known as levothyroxine or L-thyroxin, is most commonly prescribed for the treatment of hypothyroidism.

MATCHING

Match each drug to its pharmacological classification. _____

1. _____ Armour 60 mg (United States)   A. thioamides

2. _____ Cytomel 50 mcg   B. synthetic T_3

3. _____ methimazole 5 mg   C. synthetic T_4

4. _____ levothyroxine 0.2 mg   D. desiccated thyroid

TRUE OR FALSE

1. _____ Hyperthyroidism and hypothyroidism are more prevalent in women than in men.

2. _____ The brand name for liothyronine is Tapazole.

3. _____ Synthroid (United States)and Eltroxin (Canada) are brand names for levothyroxine.

4. _____ Cigarette smoking increases the risk for developing thyroid-related eye disease.

5. _____ A low TSH level signals hypothyroidism.

6. _____ Free T_4 index (FT4I) or FT4 levels are high when hyperthyroidism is present.

7. _____ Pharmacy technicians should attempt to dispense the same manufacturer's product of levothyroxine each time the patient's prescription is refilled.

CRITICAL THINKING

The following hard copy is brought to your pharmacy for filling. Identify the prescription error(s). (You already have patient's full address on file.)

Anh Dang Tu, MD   Date _____
1421 Rainier S
Anytown, USA

Pt. Name _____ Howard Dean _____
Address _____

℞ Synthroid 100mg tablet   #30
    1 tab daily

Refills _____

_____   _____ AD Tu _____
Substitution permitted   Dispense as written

---

1. Spot the error in the following prescription:

   _____

   A. Quantity missing
   B. Directions incomplete
   C. Strength missing
   D. Strength incorrect
   E. Dosage form missing

Kathy Principi, MD   Date _____
1145 Broadway
Anytown, USA

Pt. Name _____ Wilma Jones _____
Address _____

℞ l-thyroxin 25mcg #30   1 tablet daily
    Prenatal vitamins with Fe #100
    1 tablet daily with food

Refills _____

    Principi   _____
Substitution permitted   Dispense as written

---

2. Wilma Jones brings the following prescriptions to your pharmacy. Why must you consult with the pharmacist before filling the prescriptions? What concerns might the pharmacist have with the prescriptions as written?

   _____

   _____

   _____

   _____

   _____

1. Pharmacy technicians should attempt to dispense the same manufacturer's product each time the patient's prescription for natural and synthetic thyroid medicine is refilled. Why is this advice given?

   _____

   _____

   _____

   _____

   _____

33 Treatment of Diabetes Mellitus

FILL IN THE BLANK

Match each term with the correct definition below. Some terms may not be used.

A. Diabetes mellitus

B. Diabetic neuropathy

C. Fasting blood glucose

D. Gestational diabetes

E. Hemoglobin A1c (Hb$_{A1c}$)

F. Hyperglycemia

G. Hypoglycemia

H. Insulin resistance

I. Prediabetes

J. Triglyceride

K. Type 1 diabetes

L. Type 2 diabetes

M. Postprandial

1. A person who has developed _____ may experience symptoms of pain or loss of feeling in the toes, feet, legs, hands, or arms.

2. Diabetes mellitus produces _____ (elevated blood glucose levels).

3. An adverse effect to sulfonylurea drugs is _____ (decreased blood glucose levels).

4. _____ is a condition of impaired fasting glucose (IFG) and impaired glucose tolerance (IGT) in which the body consistently has high normal glucose levels.

5. _____ may be caused by the hormones of pregnancy or a shortage of insulin.

6. Whereas a person with _____ produces little or no insulin, _____ is a condition in which the pancreas produce a sufficient amount of insulin but insulin receptors lack sensitivity to the insulin produced.

7. A precursor to type 2 diabetes, known as _____, is a condition in which the body does not respond to insulin.

8. High _____ levels in the blood may raise the risks for heart attack or stroke.

9. A(n) _____ test is taken after a person has not eaten for 8 to 12 hours.

10. _____ is a chronic condition in which the body is unable to properly convert food into energy.

11. The _____ blood test measures a person's average blood glucose level over a period of weeks or months.

12. _____ is a term that means after eating.

MULTIPLE CHOICE

1. Select the **false** statement. _____
   A. Diabetes is the seventh leading cause of death in Canada.
   B. Diabetes is the leading cause of non–war-related amputations.
   C. Diabetes is the leading cause of death in the United States.
   D. Glucose in the bloodstream leaves a sticky residue over all the body's organs and cells, causing damage.
   E. Diabetes mellitus is a disorder of metabolism that involves glucose utilization.

2. Select the **false** statement. _____
   A. Insulin is released by the beta cells in the islets of Langerhans.
   B. Insulin is only administered for the treatment of type 1 diabetes.
   C. Insulin lowers blood glucose levels.
   D. Insulin may be administered by IV infusion, insulin pump, subcutaneous injection, and inhalation therapy.

3. Select the **true** statement. _____
   A. Prediabetes causes impaired fasting glucose (IFG) and impaired glucose tolerance (IGT).
   B. In type 1 diabetes, the immune system attacks and destroys the beta cells in the pancreas so insufficient amounts of insulin are produced.
   C. In type 2 diabetes, the pancreas usually produces sufficient amounts of insulin but is unable to use the insulin effectively.
   D. Gestational diabetes may be caused by the hormones of pregnancy or a shortage of insulin.
   E. All of the above are true.

4. Elevated glucose levels may be measured by

   _____.
   A. urine glucose testing
   B. blood glucose monitoring
   C. hemoglobin A1c (Hb_{A1c}) test
   D. all of the above

5. All of the following agents stimulate insulin secretion from beta cells in the pancreas *except*

   _____.
   A. meglitinides
   B. miglitol
   C. sulfonylureas

6. All of the following agents are administered orally to

   treat type 2 diabetes *except* _____.
   A. glimepiride
   B. insulin
   C. miglitol
   D. sitagliptin
   E. metformin

FILL IN THE BLANK: DRUG NAMES

1. What is the *generic name* for Humalog? _____

2. What is the *brand name* for insulin glargine? _____

3. What is the *brand name* for glyburide (United States) and glibenclamide (Canada)? _____

4. What is the *generic name* for Amaryl? _____

5. What is the *generic name* for Glucophage? _____

6. What are the *brand names* for acarbose? _____

7. What is the *generic name* for Starlix? _____

8. What is the *brand name* for repaglinide? _____

9. What is the *generic name* for Actos? _____

10. What is the *generic name* for Avandia? _____

11. What is the *brand name* for rosiglitazone + glimepiride? _____

12. What is the *generic name* for Januvia (United States)? _____

13. What is the *generic name* for Byetta (United States)? _____

14. What is the *brand name* for pramlintide? _____

MATCHING

Match each drug to its pharmacological classification.

1. _____ Amaryl 2 mg	A. thiazolidinediones
2. _____ acarbose 50 mg	B. meglitinides
3. _____ rosiglitazone 2 mg	C. alpha glucosidase inhibitors
4. _____ nateglinide120 mg	D. biguanides
5. _____ Glucophage 750 mg XR	E. sulfonylureas

MATCHING

Patient education is an essential component of therapeutics. Select the best warning label to apply to the prescription vial given to patients taking the drugs listed.

1. _____ pioglitazone	A. REFRIGERATE; DO NOT FREEZE
2. _____ Starlix	B. TAKE WITH THE FIRST BITE OF A MEAL
3. _____ acarbose	C. AVOID ALCOHOL
4. _____ Humalog	D. SWALLOW TABLETS WITH WATER; DO NOT CHEW

TRUE OR FALSE

1. _____ A common ending for thiazolidinediones is *-glitazone*.

2. _____ Extended release dosage forms of metformin are substitutable.

3. _____ Pramlintide can be mixed with other injectables, including insulin.

4. _____ A common ending for meglitinides is *-glinide*.

5. _____ Conventional and micronized dosage forms of glyburide are not substitutable.

6. _____ Acarbose and miglitol must be administered with the first bite of each meal.

CRITICAL THINKING

1. Complete the table and categorize insulin according to its onset and duration of action.

ULTRA RAPID	RAPID	INTERMEDIATE	LONG

2. During a serious infection, Mr. Perkins is switched to insulin therapy: Humalog 15 units QAM and Humulin N 20 units QAM. How many days will each of the 10-mL insulin bottles last? Please show your calculations.

_____

_____

_____

_____

_____

The following hard copies are brought to your pharmacy for filling. Identify the prescription error(s). (You already have the patient's full address on file.)

```
Anh Dang Tu, MD          Date _____
1145 Broadway
Anytown, USA

Pt. Name _____ Lili Olschefsky _____
Address _____

Rx   pioglitazone   #30
       1 tablet daily



Refills _____

_____        _____ Tu _____
Substitution permitted   Dispense as written
```

3. Spot the error in the following prescription:

   _____

   A. Quantity missing
   B. Directions incomplete
   C. Strength missing
   D. Strength incorrect
   E. Dosage form missing

```
┌─────────────────────────────────────────┐
│         Kathy Principi, MD    Date _____ │
│            1145 Broadway                  │
│            Anytown, USA                   │
│                                           │
│  Pt. Name _____ Will Jones _____  │
│  Address _____  │
│  ℞   Amaryl 2mg                           │
│        4 mg once daily. May increase up to a maximum of │
│        8mg/day as directed                │
│                                           │
│  Refills _____                           │
│                                           │
│  _____Principi_____      _____  │
│  Substitution permitted  Dispense as written │
└─────────────────────────────────────────┘
```

4. Spot the error in the following prescription:

_____

A. Quantity missing

B. Directions incomplete

C. Strength missing

D. Strength incorrect

E. Dosage form missing

RESEARCH ACTIVITY

Access the National Library of Medicine's website (http://www.nlm.nih.gov/medlineplus/) to answer the following questions.

1. Why might individuals with type 1 and type 2 diabetes benefit from making lifestyle changes? Identify recommended changes and discuss the role of nutritional supplements.

_____

_____

_____

_____

_____

2. Why might individuals with type 2 diabetes be advised to monitor their blood glucose levels daily?

_____

_____

_____

_____

_____

34 Drugs That Affect the Reproductive System

FILL IN THE BLANK

Match each term with the correct definition below. Some terms may not be used.

A. Amenorrhea

B. Condom

C. Diaphragm

D. Fertility

E. Hypogonadism

F. Hysterectomy

G. Infertility

H. Kallmann syndrome

I. Klinefelter syndrome

J. Menopause

K. Menorrhagia

L. Premenstrual dysphoric disorder

M. Premenstrual syndrome

N. Prolactinoma

O. Endometriosis

P. Dysmenorrhea

Q. Atrophic vaginitis

R. Craniopharyngioma

S. Dysfunctional uterine bleeding

T. Intrauterine device

U. Osteoporosis

V. Pelvic inflammatory disease

W. Polycystic ovary disease

X. Pregnancy

Y. Salpingitis

Z. Supraovulation

AA. Toxic shock syndrome (TSS)

BB. Turner syndrome

CC. Vaginitis

1. _____ is a pituitary tumor that produces excessive amount of prolactin.

2. _____ is excessive menstrual bleeding; the opposite is _____, the absence of normal menstruation.

3. The _____ is a rubber or plastic cup that fits over the cervix and is used for contraceptive purposes.

4. The medical term for surgical removal of the uterus is _____.

5. _____ and _____ are related conditions that have symptoms such as depression, anxiety, or irritability and are linked to the menstrual cycle.

6. _____ is the quality of being productive or able to become pregnant; the opposite is

   _____, an inability to achieve pregnancy during 1 year or more of unprotected intercourse.

7. A _____ is a contraceptive device that fits over the penile sheath and is made of synthetic or natural materials.

8. _____. is a condition in which functioning endometrial tissue is located outside the uterus.

   The condition may cause _____ (difficult or painful menstruation).

9. _____ is a condition in which there is an inadequate production of sex hormones.

10. Congenital disorders linked to the male reproductive system are _____ (causes hypogonadism)

    and _____ (marked by primary testicular failure).

11. The definition of _____ is the termination of menstrual cycles.

12. _____ is irregular or excessive uterine bleeding that results either from a structural problem or hormonal imbalance.

13. _____ is the loss of bone mass that occurs throughout the skeleton, predisposing patients to fractures.

14. _____ is inflammation of the fallopian tube, usually as a result of a sexually transmitted disease (STD).

15. Inflammation of the vagina is known as _____.

16. _____ is a rare disorder caused by certain *Staphylococcus aureus* strains seen in women using tampons.

17. _____ is the simultaneous rupture of multiple mature follicles.

18. Postmenopausal thinning and dryness of the vaginal epithelium related to decreased estrogen levels is known as _____.

19. _____ is a pituitary tumor that causes hormonal deficiencies.

20. _____ is a condition that is characterized by ovaries twice the normal size that are studded with fluid-filled cysts.

21. _____ is a device inserted in the uterus to prevent pregnancy.

22. The condition of having a developing embryo or fetus in the body after successful conception is known as _____.

23. _____ is a congenital endocrine disorder caused by a failure of the ovaries to respond to pituitary hormone (gonadotropin) stimulation.

24. _____ is an infection of the uterus, fallopian tubes, and adjacent pelvic structures that is not associated with pregnancy or surgery.

MULTIPLE CHOICE

1. Which of the following is *not* an effective method of birth control? _____
   A. foam and condom
   B. diaphragm and spermicide
   C. withdrawal
   D. oral contraceptives
   E. IUD

2. The diaphragm must be inserted sometime before sexual intercourse and should remain in the vagina for_____ after a man's last ejaculation.
   A. 1 to 2 hours
   B. 3 to 4 hours
   C. 5 to 6 hours
   D. 6 to 8 hours

3. Which of the following methods of contraception can prevent sexually transmitted infections such as HIV and syphilis? _____
   A. oral contraceptives
   B. IUD
   C. diaphragm
   D. condoms

4. Emergency contraceptives (Plan B) must be taken _____ of unprotected intercourse.
   A. within 1 to 2 hours
   B. within 3 to 6 hours
   C. within 24 hours
   D. within 72 hours
   E. within 1 week

5. Standard penicillins (e.g., penicillin G and ampicillin) lack stability in gastric acids, which is why most are administered _____.
   A. on an empty stomach
   B. with food
   C. with a full meal
   D. sublingually

6. Select the pair of drugs that are used for the treatment of a *Chlamydia* infection. _____
   A. azithromycin and doxycycline
   B. clarithromycin and erythromycin
   C. ciprofloxacin and cefixime
   D. tetracycline and erythromycin

FILL IN THE BLANK: DRUG NAMES

1. What is the ***brand name*** for ethinyl estradiol + drospirenone ? _____

2. What is the ***generic name*** for Alesse (United States) and Min-Ovral (Canada)? _____

3. What is the ***brand name*** for ethinyl estradiol + etonogestrel? _____

4. What is the ***generic name*** for Plan B? _____

5. What are **brand names** for progesterone (progestin)? _____

6. What is the **generic name** for Premarin? _____

7. What is a **brand name** for esterified estrogen? _____

8. What is the **generic name** for conjugated estrogens + medroxyprogesterone acetate? _____

9. What are **brand name**s for clomiphene? _____

10. What is the **generic name** for Androderm? _____

11. What is the **brand name** for goserelin? _____

12. What is the **generic name** for Synarel? _____

13. What are **brand names** for Leuprolide? _____

MATCHING

Match each drug to its pharmacological family.

1. _____ Lupron 3.75 mg   A. estrogen

2. _____ Clomid 50 mg   B. progestin

3. _____ Androderm 2.5 mg/hr   C. antiestrogen

4. _____ Crinone vaginal gel   D. gonadotropin-releasing hormone

5. _____ Estrace 2 mg   E. androgen

MATCHING

Match each drug to its therapeutic use.

1. _____ danazol 100 mg   A. infertility

2. _____ FemHRT   B. endometriosis

3. _____ Clomid 50 mg   C. hypogonadism

4. _____ Yasmin   D. oral contraceptive

5. _____ testosterone   E. hormone replacement therapy

TRUE OR FALSE

1. _____ A common ending of androgen agonists is *-sterone*.

2. _____ Testosterone patches are *not* substitutable.

3. _____ Testosterone and other anabolic steroids are controlled substances in the United States.

4. _____ Vivelle and Vivelle dot patches are substitutable.

5. _____ The Women's Health Initiative (WHI) led physicians to increase prescribing of hormone replacement therapy (HRT).

CRITICAL THINKING

The following hard copies are brought to your pharmacy for filling. Identify the prescription error(s). (You already have the patient's full address on file.)

Anh Dang Tu, MD   Date _____
1145 Broadway
Anytown, USA

Pt. Name _____ Lili Olschefsky _____
Address _____

℞   *Nuva-Ring*

    insert one ring vaginally daily

Refills _____

_____   *Tu* _____

Substitution permitted   Dispense as written

---

1. Spot the error in the following prescription:

    _____

    A. Quantity missing
    B. Directions incorrect
    C. Strength missing
    D. Strength incorrect
    E. Dosage form missing

Kathy Principi, MD   Date _____
1145 Broadway
Anytown, USA

Pt. Name _____ Will Jones _____
Address _____

℞   *clomiphene 50mg*   *#5*

    Take 1 tablet daily on day 5-10 of menstrual cycle

Refills _____

_____ *Principi* _____   _____

Substitution permitted   Dispense as written

---

2. Spot the error in the following prescription:

    _____

    A. Quantity missing
    B. Directions incomplete
    C. Strength missing
    D. Strength incorrect
    E. Verify prescription is written for correct patient

RESEARCH ACTIVITY

1. Anabolic steroids are controlled substances to reduce abuse. Identify health problems that are linked to abuse. Access the National Library of Medicine's website (http://www.nlm.nih.gov/medlineplus/anabolicsteroids.html) to answer the question.

    _____

    _____

    _____

    _____

    _____

35 Treatment of Bacterial Infection

TERMS AND DEFINITIONS

Match each term with the correct definition below. Some terms may not be used.

A. Antibiotic

B. β-Lactamase

C. Bactericidal

D. Bacteriostatic

E. Microbial resistance

F. Antimicrobial

G. Broad-spectrum antibiotic

H. Deoxyribonucleic acid (DNA)

I. Ribonucleic acid (RNA)

1. Whereas antiinfective agents that are able to destroy bacteria are _____, antiinfective agents that are _____ inhibit bacterial proliferation.

2. _____ is an enzyme secreted by some microbes that has the ability to destroy β-lactam antibiotics.

3. A natural substance produced by one organism that is capable of destroying or inhibiting the growth of bacteria is called a(n) _____.

4. The term used to describe the process of bacteria developing mechanisms to overcome the bactericidal effects of an antibiotic is _____.

5. Nucleic acids involved in protein synthesis that carry and transfer genetic information and assemble proteins are known as _____.

6. _____ is a substance capable of destroying or inhibiting the growth of a microorganisms.

7. An antimicrobial that is capable of destroying a wide range of bacteria is a(n) _____.

8. _____ is the nucleic acids that contain the genetic blue print.

MATCHING

1. A common ending for aminoglycoside family of antiinfectives is _____.

2. A common ending for fluoroquinolone family of antiinfectives is _____.

3. A common beginning for cephalosporin family of antiinfectives is _____.

4. A common ending for macrolide family of antiinfectives is _____.

5. A common ending for penicillin family antiinfectives is _____.

6. A common beginning for sulfonamides family of antiinfectives is _____.

7. A common ending for tetracycline family antiinfectives is _____.

A. *-ceph* or *cef*

B. *-sulf*

C. *-thromycin*

D. *-mycin* or *micin*

E. *-cycline*

F. *-cillin*

G. *-floxacin*

MULTIPLE CHOICE

1. Select the **false** statement. _____
   A. Poverty, malnutrition, and lack of clean water increase the risk for infectious disease.
   B. Poor sanitation and inadequate housing increase the risk for infectious disease.
   C. Infectious disease is no longer a leading cause of morbidity and mortality globally.
   D. Antibiotics have played a key role in improving the survival of individuals with bacterial infections.

2. Select the **false** statement about microbial resistance. _____
   A. It can result in new "super bugs" that are resistant to currently available antiinfective agents.
   B. It cannot be transferred to other bacteria.
   C. It can be caused by failure to complete the full course of therapy.
   D. It can be caused by inappropriate prescribing.

3. Causes of microbial resistance are _____.
   A. administration of antibacterial agents for viral infections (e.g., the common cold)
   B. antibiotics in the food chain (agriculture, animal husbandry, fish farms)
   C. lack of guidelines for preventing spread of infections in institutional care settings
   D. all of the above

4. β-Lactam antibiotics target the bacterial cell wall. All of the following drugs are β-lactam antibiotics *except* _____.
   A. penicillins
   B. erythromycin
   C. cephalosporins
   D. carbapenems
   E. monobactams

5. Some penicillins (e.g., penicillin G and ampicillin) lack stability in gastric acids, which is why most are administered _____.
   A. on an empty stomach
   B. with food
   C. with a full meal
   D. sublingually

6. Select the **false** statement. _____
   A. Cephalosporins may be classified as first, second, third, fourth, and fifth generation.
   B. Clarithromycin is a key ingredient in treatment regimens for peptic ulcer disease caused by the bacteria *H. pylori*.
   C. Gastrointestinal upset is a common adverse reaction that occurs with erythromycin.
   D. Sulfonamides may be used to treat AIDS-related pneumonia (*Pneumocystis carinii*).

FILL IN THE BLANK: DRUG NAMES

1. What is the ***brand name*** for cephalexin? _____

2. What is the ***generic name*** for Ciloxan? _____

3. What are ***brand name***s for erythromycin base (delayed release)? _____

4. What is the ***generic name*** for Levaquin? _____

5. What is the **brand name** for clarithromycin? _____

6. What is the **generic name** for Zithromax? _____

7. What is a **brand name** for minocycline? _____

8. What is the **generic name** for Vibramycin? _____

9. What is a **brand name** for sulfamethoxazole + trimethoprim? _____

10. What is the **generic name** for Bactroban? _____

11. What is the **generic name** for Cleocin? _____

12. What is a **brand name** for sulfamethoxazole + erythromycin ethylsuccinate? _____

MATCHING

Match each drug to its pharmacological family.

1. _____ tobramycin 0.3% OS   A. tetracycline family

2. _____ cephalexin 250 mg cap   B. sulfonamide family

3. _____ amoxicillin 250 mg/5 mL   C. cephalosporin family

4. _____ Minocin 100 mg cap   D. aminoglycoside family

5. _____ sulfadiazine cream 1%   E. penicillin family

MATCHING

Match each drug to its therapeutic use.

1. _____ isoniazid 300 mg   A. acne rosacea

2. _____ Bactroban ointment   B. tuberculosis

3. _____ metronidazole topical gel   C. bacterial meningitis

4. _____ clindamycin 150 mg cap   D. pseudomembranous colitis

5. _____ chloramphenicol   E. impetigo

TRUE OR FALSE

1. _____ The warning label TAKE WITH LOTS OF WATER is applied to prescription vials for sulfonamides.

2. _____ Oral and parenteral fluoroquinolones are contraindicated in pregnant women and people older than 16 to 18 years.

3. _____ Persons who are allergic to penicillin may also be allergic to cephalosporins.

4. _____ Tetracyclines are contraindicated in pregnancy and small children because they can weaken fetal bone, retard bone growth, weaken tooth enamel, and stain teeth.

5. _____ The milligram strength of clavulanic acid is the same for all strengths and dosage forms of Augmentin (United States) and Clavulin (Canada).

6. _____ SMX-TMP is an abbreviation for Pediazole.

7. _____ Macrolides and penicillins may decrease the effectiveness of oral contraceptives.

CRITICAL THINKING

The following hard copies are brought to your pharmacy for filling. Identify the prescription error(s). (You already have the patient's full address on file.)

Anh Dang Tu, MD   Date _____
1145 Broadway
Anytown, USA

Pt. Name _____ Lili Olschefsky _____

Address _____

Rx   amoxicillin + clavulanic acid tablet   #30

    i TID

Refills _____

_____   Tu _____

Substitution permitted   Dispense as written

1. Spot the error in the following prescription:

_____

A. Quantity missing

B. Directions incomplete

C. Strength missing

D. Strength incorrect

E. Dosage form missing

Kathy Principi, MD   Date _____
1145 Broadway
Anytown, USA

Pt. Name _____ Will Jones _____

Address _____

Rx   isoniazid 300mg

    900mg/day twice weekly with pyridoxine

Refills _____

_____ Principi _____

Substitution permitted   Dispense as written

2. Spot the error in the following prescription:

_____

A. Quantity missing

B. Directions incomplete

C. Strength missing

D. Strength incorrect

E. Dosage form missing

Kathy Principi, MD   Date _____
1145 Broadway
Anytown, USA

Pt. Name _____ Ellen Wilber _____

Address _____

Rx   clarithromycin 250mg

    Take 2 tablets on day 1st day; then take one tablet

    daily on days 2 thru 5.

Refills _____

_____ Principi _____

Substitution permitted   Dispense as written

3. Spot the error in the following prescription:

_____

A. Quantity missing

B. Directions incomplete

C. Strength missing

D. Strength incorrect

E. Drug possibly incorrect; verify

```
┌─────────────────────────────────────────┐
│          Kathy Principi, MD    Date _____ │
│             1145 Broadway                 │
│             Anytown, USA                  │
│                                           │
│  Pt. Name _____ Preston Scott _____ │
│  Address _____ │
│                                           │
│  ℞   SMX-TMP DS capsule    #30            │
│         i tab BID                         │
│                                           │
│                                           │
│  Refills _____                           │
│       Principi                            │
│  _____    _____ │
│  Substitution permitted   Dispense as written │
└─────────────────────────────────────────┘
```

4. Spot the error in the following prescription:

   _____

   A. Quantity missing
   B. Directions incomplete
   C. Strength missing
   D. Strength incorrect
   E. Dosage form incorrect

RESEARCH ACTIVITY

Access the National Library of Medicine's website (http://www.nlm.nih.gov/medlineplus/antibiotics.html) to answer the following questions.

1. What causes antimicrobial resistance?

   _____

   _____

   _____

   _____

   _____

2. What role can the pharmacist and pharmacy technician play in helping patients reduce the risk of developing resistance?

   _____

   _____

   _____

   _____

   _____

36 Treatment of Viral Infections

TERMS AND DEFINITIONS

Match each term with the correct definition below. Some terms may not be used.

A. AIDS (acquired immune deficiency syndrome)

B. Antiretroviral

C. Antiviral

D. Antiviral resistance

E. CD4 T lymphocyte

F. Cross-resistance

G. Drug resistance testing

H. Host

I. Viral load

J. Virion

K. Virostatic

L. Virus

M. Adherence

N. CD4 count

O. Highly active antiretroviral therapy

P. Mother-to-child transmission

Q. Oncovirus

1. _____ is a laboratory test to determine if an individual's HIV strain is resistant to any anti-HIV medications.

2. The infectious particles of a virus are called _____.

3. A virus may develop _____, an ability to overcome the suppressive action of an antiviral agent.

4. The _____ is the amount of materials from the virus that get released into the blood when the HIV virus reproduces.

5. An individual who is infected with a virus is called a(n) _____.

6. A(n) _____ antiviral agent is able to suppress viral proliferation.

7. _____ is a type of white blood cell that fights infection.

8. _____ is the most severe form of HIV infection.

9. A(n) _____ is an intracellular parasite that consists of a DNA and RNA core surrounded by a protein coat and sometimes an outer covering of lipoprotein.

10. A virus may develop _____, resistance to multiple drugs in a particular drug classification.

11. A(n) _____ is an medication that inhibits with the replication of retroviruses.

12. _____ is a combination of three or more antiretroviral medications taken in a regimen.

13. Transmission of the HIV from an HIV-infected mother to her baby during pregnancy or delivery or through breast milk is known as _____.

14. _____ is closely following or adhering to the treatment regimen.

15. _____ is a virus that is an etiologic agent in a cancer.

16. The number of CD4 cells in a sample of blood is the _____.

MATCHING

1. A common ending for antivirals that inhibit viral uncoating is _____.

2. A common ending for antivirals used for the treatment of herpes virus infections is _____.

3. A common ending for protease inhibitors is _____.

4. A common ending for neuramidase inhibitors is _____.

A. *-cyclovir* and *-ciclovir*

B. *-navir*

C. *-mantadine*

D. *-amivir*

MULTIPLE CHOICE

1. HIV-infected patients are diagnosed with AIDS when their CD4 cell count falls below _____ or if they develop an AIDS-defining illness.
   A. 200 cells/mm^3
   B. 300 cells/mm^3
   C. 400 cells/mm^3
   D. 600 cells/mm^3

2. Perinatal mother-to-child transmission of the HIV virus from an HIV-infected mother to her baby can occur _____.
   A. during pregnancy
   B. delivery
   C. through breastfeeding
   D. all of the above

3. Highly active antiretroviral therapy (HAART) is a treatment regimen for the treatment of HIV/AIDS that consists of _____.
   A. one antiretroviral drug
   B. one or two antiretroviral drugs
   C. two or three antiretroviral drugs
   D. three or more antiretroviral drugs

4. The risk of perinatal mother-to-child transmission of HIV may be reduced by the administration of a dose of _____ to the mother during delivery and to the baby upon birth or zidovudine only.
   A. zidovudine + nevirapine
   B. abacavir + zidovudine
   C. tenofovir + zidovudine
   D. Sustiva + zidovudine

5. A virus that is linked to cervical cancer is

_____.
   A. cold sores
   B. human papillomavirus (HPV)
   C. HIV
   D. herpes zoster

6. The NRTI that may be administered as monotherapy for the prevention of mother-to-child transmission

   (PMTCT) of HIV is _____.
   A. Zidovudine
   B. ganciclovir
   C. emtricitabine
   D. Sustiva

7. Select the **false** statement. _____
   A. Antivirals are only effective against a specific virus.
   B. Antibiotics are effective against viral infections.
   C. Viruses continually mutate making it difficult to develop a vaccine to prevent virus infection.
   D. Antivirals inhibit virus-specific steps in the replication cycle.

8. Which drug is *not* prescribed for the treatment of

cytomegalovirus retinitis? _____
   A. cidofovir
   B. saquinavir
   C. foscarnet
   D. ganciclovir

9. The steps in the HIV life cycle are _____.
   A. binding, fusion, and uncoating
   B. reverse transcription and integration
   C. genome replication and protein synthesis
   D. protein cleavage, assembly, and virus release
   E. all of the above

10. Nevirapine is associated with fatal

_____ toxicity, and the FDA has required changes in the package labeling to warn of this adverse effect.
   A. kidney
   B. heart
   C. liver
   D. thyroid

FILL IN THE BLANK: DRUG NAMES

1. What is the ***brand name*** for amantadine? _____

2. What is the ***generic name*** for Flumadine (United States)? _____

3. What is the ***generic name*** for Tamiflu? _____

4. What is the ***generic name*** for Relenza? _____

5. What is the ***brand name*** for interferon alfacon-1? _____

6. What is the ***generic name*** for Pegasys? _____

7. What is the ***brand name*** for acyclovir? _____

8. What is the ***generic name*** for PEG-intron (United States) and Pegetron (Canada)? _____

9. What is the ***generic name*** for Famvir? _____

10. What is the ***generic name*** for Foscavir (United States)? _____

11. What is the ***brand name*** for ganciclovir? _____

12. What is the ***brand name*** for penciclovir? _____

13. What is the ***generic name*** for Viroptic? _____

14. What is the ***generic name*** for Valtrex? _____

15. What is the ***generic name*** for Valcyte (Canada)? _____

16. What is the *generic name* for Virazole? _____

17. What is the *brand name* for abacavir? _____

18. What is the *brand name* for didanosine? _____

19. What is the *generic name* for Emtriva? _____

20. What is the *generic name* for Epivir? _____

21. What is the *brand name* for stavudine? _____

22. What is the *brand name* for tenofovir DF? _____

23. What is the *generic name* for Retrovir? _____

24. What is the *generic name* for Truvada? _____

25. What is the *brand name* for abacavir + lamivudine + zidovudine? _____

26. What is the *generic name* for Epzicom (United States) and Kivexa (Canada)? _____

27. What is the *brand name* for delavirdine? _____

28. What is the *generic name* for lamivudine + zidovudine? _____

29. What is the *brand name* for efavirenz? _____

30. What is the *generic name* for Atripla (United States)? _____

31. What is the *brand name* for nevirapine? _____

32. What is the *generic name* for Agenerase? _____

33. What is the *brand name* for atazanavir? _____

34. What is the *generic name* for Prezista? _____

35. What is the *brand name* for indinavir? _____

36. What is the *generic name* for Lexiva (United States) and Telzir (Canada)? _____

37. What is the *brand name* for nelfinavir? _____

38. What is the *brand name* for ritonavir? _____

39. What is the *brand name* for saquinavir? _____

40. What is the *generic name* for Aptivus? _____

41. What is the *brand name* for lopinavir + ritonavir? _____

42. What is the *generic name* for Fuzeon? _____

MATCHING

Match each drug to its pharmacological family.

1. _____ acyclovir

2. _____ Tamiflu

3. _____ Intron-A

4. _____ amantadine

A. inhibitor of viral uncoating

B. neuraminidase inhibitor

C. interferon

D. inhibition of DNA and RNA replication

MATCHING

Match each drug to its therapeutic use.

1. _____ peginterferon alfa-2b

2. _____ Tamiflu

3. _____ Virazole

4. _____ Cytovene

5. _____ penciclovir

A. herpes

B. influenza

C. hepatitis C

D. RSV

E. cytomegalovirus (CMV)

MATCHING

Match each drug to its pharmacological family.

1. _____ nevirapine

2. _____ Fuzeon

3. _____ Norvir

4. _____ lamivudine

A. nucleoside and nucleotide reverse transcriptase inhibitors (NRTIs)

B. non-nucleoside reverse transcriptase inhibitors (NNRTIs)

C. protease inhibitor

D. fusion inhibitor

CRITICAL THINKING

The following hard copies are brought to your pharmacy for filling. Identify the prescription error(s). (You already have the patient's full address on file.)

Kathy Principi, MD
1145 Broadway
Anytown, USA

Date *1-28-05*

Pt. Name _____ Ellen Wilber _____

Address _____

℞ *Videx oral solution 10mg/ml*
    12ml BID

Refills _____

_____ *Principi* _____   _____

Substitution permitted   Dispense as written

1. Spot the error in the following prescription:

   _____

   A. Quantity missing
   B. Directions incomplete
   C. Strength missing
   D. Strength incorrect
   E. Dosage form incorrect

```
           Kathy Principi, MD        Date 1-28-05
              1145 Broadway
              Anytown, USA

Pt. Name _____ Ellen Wilber _____
Address _____
Rx    Tamiflu 12mg/ml   25ml
      BID x 5 days



Refills _____
_____Principi_____        _____
Substitution permitted       Dispense as written
```

2. Spot the error in the following prescription:

_____

A. Quantity missing

B. Directions incomplete

C. Strength missing

D. Strength incorrect

E. Dosage form incorrect

3. Give four pairs of drug names that have look-alike or sound-alike issues with drugs used for neuromuscular blockade.

DRUG NAME	LOOK-ALIKE OR SOUND-ALIKE DRUG

RESEARCH ACTIVITY

Access the Merck Manual Online's website (http://www.merck.com/mmpe/sec14/ch188/ch188d.html#sec14-ch188 -ch188d-2325), the Centers for Disease Control and Prevention's website (http://www.cdc.gov), and other websites to complete the research activity.

1. What is a flu pandemic, and what is its cause?

_____

_____

_____

_____

_____

2. How do scientists determine which strain(s) of flu to create a vaccine for?

_____

_____

_____

_____

_____

37 Treatment of Cancers

TERMS AND DEFINITIONS

Match each term with the correct definition below. Some terms may not be used.

A. Benign

B. Biopsy

C. Double-contrast barium enema

D. Leukemia

E. Lymphoma

F. Mammography

G. Metastasis

H. Neoplasm

I. Positron emission tomography (PET) scan

J. Radionuclide scan

K. Sonography

L. Stem cell

M. Stem cell transplantation

N. Tumor

O. Chemotherapy

P. Complementary and alternative medicine (CAM)

Q. Computed tomography (CT) scan

R. Excisional biopsy

S. External radiation

T. Fecal occult blood test (FOBT)

U. Implant radiation

V. Ionizing radiation

W. Malignant

X. Oncovirus

Y. Pap test or Pap smear

Z. Polyp

AA. Primary tumor

BB. Prostate-specific antigen (PSA) test

CC. Radiation therapy

DD. Radon

EE. Stage

FF. Tumor marker

GG. Cancer

HH. Melanoma

1. A(n) _____ is a computer picture of internal organs and tissues produced by ultrasound.

2. A tumor that is not cancerous is _____ and does not spread to surrounding tissues or other parts of the body.

3. _____ is a diagnostic examination the uses radioactive glucose (sugar).

4. The colon and rectum may be examined for signs of cancer by administering a _____ and then taking radiographs of the area.

5. _____ is a type of cell from which other types of cells develop and that may be administered to replace cells that have been damaged by cancer treatment in a process called _____.

6. A cancer that begins in cells of the immune system is called a(n) _____.

7. A(n) _____ is taken using a scanner that can take pictures of the internal parts of the body and detect where the radiation concentrates.

8. A(n) _____ is a screening examination to detect breast cancer.

9. A(n) _____, the removal of cells for examination by a pathologist, may be performed to determine whether a(n) _____ or _____ (mass of excess tissue that results from abnormal cell division) is benign or malignant.

10. _____ is a cancer that starts in blood-forming tissue such as the bone marrow.

11. The spread of cancer from one part of the body to another is called _____.

12. _____ is the extent of a cancer within the body. Staging is based on the size of the tumor, whether lymph nodes contain cancer, and whether the disease has spread from the original site to other parts of the body.

13. _____ is a test that measures level of free PSA, a protein produced by the prostate gland. Levels are elevated in men who have prostate cancer, infection, or inflammation of the prostate gland and BPH.

14. Cancerous tumors that can invade and destroy nearby tissue and spread to other parts of the body are considered to be _____.

15. _____ is a test to check for blood in stool.

16. Treatment with drugs that kill cancer is known as _____.

17. _____ is a term for diseases in which abnormal cells divide without control.

18. _____ is a surgical procedure in which an entire lump of suspicious-looking tissue is removed for diagnosis.

19. _____ is a virus that is an etiologic agent in a cancer.

20. _____ or _____ is a screening test in which cells from the cervix are examined to detect cancer and changes that may lead to cancer.

21. Treatments that may include dietary supplements, herbal preparations, acupuncture, massage, magnet therapy, spiritual healing, and meditation are known as _____.

22. _____ is radiation therapy that uses a machine to aim high-energy rays at the cancer.

23. _____ is a growth that protrudes from a mucous membrane.

24. Substance sometimes found in the blood, other body fluids, or tissues that may signal the presence of a certain type of cancer is known as _____.

25. _____ is a procedure, also known as brachytherapy, in which radioactive material sealed in needles, seeds, wires, or catheters is placed directly into or near a tumor.

26. _____ is a diagnostic examination in which a series of detailed pictures are taken of areas inside the body that are created by a computer that is linked to an x-ray machine.

27. _____ is a type of high-frequency radiation produced by x-ray procedures, radioactive substances, and UV light that can lead to health risks, including cancer, at certain doses.

28. The original tumor or initial tumor is also known as the _____.

29. _____ is a radioactive gas that if inhaled in sufficient quantity can lead to lung cancer.

30. _____ uses high-energy radiation from x-rays, gamma rays, neutrons, and other sources to kill cancer cells and shrink tumors.

31. _____ is a form of skin cancer that arises in melanocytes, the cells that produce pigment.

32. _____ is another word for tumor.

33. _____ is a procedure used to replace cells that were destroyed by cancer treatment.

34. _____ is a mass of excess tissue that results from abnormal cell division.

MULTIPLE CHOICE

1. A Pap test is a screening examination for

   _____.
   A. breast cancer
   B. bladder cancer
   C. cervical cancer
   D. lung cancer

2. All of the following screening tests involve imaging

   using radioactive materials *except* _____.
   A. sonography
   B. mammography
   C. radionuclide scan
   D. positron emission tomography (PET) scan
   E. computed tomography (CT) scan

3. Cancers are categorized by stage. Staging is based on

   all of the following *except* _____.
   A. size of the tumor
   B. lymph node involvement
   C. metastasis
   D. length of time cancer has been present

4. Which source of ionizing radiation is *not* used for
   treatment of cancers?
   A. x-rays
   B. gamma rays
   C. neutrons
   D. UV light

5. A cancer that arises in the cells that produce pigment

   in the skin is called _____.
   A. melanoma
   B. lymphoma
   C. leukemia

6. Which treatment would *not* be classified as complementary and alternative medicine (CAM)?

   _____
   A. dietary supplements and herbal preparations
   B. acupuncture and massage
   C. magnet therapy
   D. chemotherapy
   E. spiritual healing and meditation

7. A warning label that is commonly affixed to most
   prescriptions for orally administered chemotherapeutic

   agents for women is _____.
   A. AVOID PREGNANCY
   B. TAKE WITH LOTS OF WATER
   C. SHAKE WELL
   D. AVOID PROLONGED SUNLIGHT

8. Select the **false** statement about lung cancer.

   _____
   A. Lung cancer is the most common form of cancer.
   B. A history of smoking tobacco is nearly always
      the cause of small cell lung cancer.
   C. Lung cancer is classified as small cell lung cancer
      and non–small cell lung cancer.
   D. Antineoplastic agents used to treat lung cancer
      are effective against both forms of the disease.

9. Which drug is *not* approved for the treatment of

   breast cancer? _____
   A. tamoxifen
   B. hydroxyurea
   C. Taxol
   D. Femara

FILL IN THE BLANK: DRUG NAMES

1. What is the ***brand name*** for fulvestrant? _____

2. What is the ***generic name*** for Soltamox (United States) and Tamofen (Canada)? _____

3. What is a ***brand name*** for exemestane? _____

4. What is the ***generic name*** for Fareston (United States)? _____

5. What is the ***generic name*** for Arimidex? _____

6. What is the ***generic name*** for Femara? _____

7. What is the ***brand name*** for goserelin? _____

8. What is the *generic name* for Megace? _____

9. What is the *generic name* for Cytoxan? _____

10. What is the *generic name* for Taxotere? _____

11. What is the *generic name* for Taxol? _____

12. What is the *brand name* vinorelbine? _____

13. What is the *generic name* for Adriamycin? _____

14. What is the *brand name* for teniposide? _____

15. What is the *generic name* for Ellence (United States) and Pharmorubicin PFS (Canada)?

_____

16. What is the *brand name* for VePesid? _____

17. What is the *generic name* for Camptosar? _____

18. What is the *brand name* for topotecan? _____

19. What is the *generic name* for Eloxatin? _____

20. What is the *generic name* for Xeloda? _____

21. What is the *generic name* for Platinol AQ (United States)? _____

22. What is the *brand name* for fludarabine? _____

23. What is the *generic name* for Paraplatin AQ (Canada)? _____

24. What is the *brand name* for cytarabine liposomal? _____

25. What is the *generic name* for Gemzar? _____

26. What is the *brand name* for pemetrexed? _____

27. What is the *generic name* for Purinethol? _____

28. What is the *generic name* for Blenoxane? _____

29. What is the *generic name* for Cosmegen? _____

30. What is the *generic name* for Hydrea? _____

MATCHING

Match each drug to its pharmacological classification.

1. _____ vincristine
2. _____ teniposide
3. _____ anastrozole
4. _____ paclitaxel
5. _____ doxorubicin

A. aromatase inhibitors
B. taxanes
C. anthracyclines
D. topoisomerase inhibitors
E. vinca alkaloid

MATCHING

Match each drug to its pharmacological classification.

1. _____ *-poside* and *-tecan*
2. _____ *-trozole*
3. _____ *-platin*
4. _____ *-rubicin*
5. _____ *-taxel*

A. aromatase inhibitors
B. taxanes
C. anthracyclines
D. topoisomerase inhibitors
E. platinum compounds

TRUE OR FALSE

1. _____ The three types of biopsy are incisional, excisional, and decisional.

2. _____ Cancerous tumors are benign.

3. _____ Specific cancers are named according to the site where the cancerous growth begins and the type of cells involved.

4. _____ Chemotherapy is treatment with drugs that kill cancer.

5. _____ Radon is radioactive gas that if inhaled in sufficient quantity can lead to lung cancer.

6. _____ A polyp is a growth that forms on the torso.

7. _____ A lymphoma is a cancer that begins in cells of the skin.

8. _____ Metastasis is the spread of cancer from one part of the body to another.

9. _____ Implant radiation is also known as brachytherapy.

10. _____ Internal radiation is a therapy that uses a machine to aim high-energy rays at the cancer.

11. _____ Doxorubicin and doxorubicin liposomal are not substitutable.

12. _____ Chemotherapeutic drugs may be prepared in a laminar flow hood.

CRITICAL THINKING

The following hard copies are brought to your pharmacy for filling. Identify the prescription error(s). (You already have the patient's full address on file.)

```
┌─────────────────────────────────────────┐
│       Anh Dang Tu, MD        Date _____ │
│       1145 Broadway                      │
│       Anytown, USA                       │
│                                          │
│ Pt. Name _____ Joan Neilsen _____ │
│ Address _____│
│ ℞   Megace   40mg/ml                     │
│     1ml QID                              │
│                                          │
│                                          │
│ Refills _____                           │
│ _____ AD Tu _____    _____ │
│ Substitution permitted   Dispense as written │
└─────────────────────────────────────────┘
```

1. Spot the error in the following prescription:

   _____

   A. Quantity missing
   B. Directions incomplete
   C. Strength missing
   D. Strength incorrect
   E. Dosage form incorrect

```
┌─────────────────────────────────────────┐
│       Anh Dang Tu, MD        Date _____ │
│       1145 Broadway                      │
│       Anytown, USA                       │
│                                          │
│ Pt. Name _____ Lili Ng _____│
│ Address _____│
│ ℞   tamoxifen   #30                      │
│     1 tab daily                          │
│                                          │
│                                          │
│ Refills _____                           │
│ _____ AD Tu _____    _____ │
│ Substitution permitted   Dispense as written │
└─────────────────────────────────────────┘
```

2. Spot the error in the following prescription:

   _____

   A. Quantity missing
   B. Directions incorrect
   C. Strength missing
   D. Strength incorrect
   E. Dosage form incorrect

3. Give six pairs of drug names that have look-alike or sound-alike issues with drugs used to treat cancer.

DRUG NAME	LOOK-ALIKE OR SOUND-ALIKE DRUG

A new vaccine has been developed to decrease the risk of cancer linked to human papillomavirus (HPV). Access the National Library of Medicine's website (http://www.nlm.nih.gov/medlineplus/healthtopics.html) and the Health Canada's website (http://www.hc-sc.gc.ca/iyh-vsv/diseases-maladies/hpv-vph_e.html) to answer the following questions about the HPV vaccine:

1. What is the trade name?

2. Who should get the vaccine?

3. When is the vaccine contraindicated?

4. What are adverse effects?

5. How effective is the vaccine?

_____

_____

_____

_____

_____

38 Vaccines, Immunomodulators, and Immunosuppressants

TERMS AND DEFINITIONS

Match each term with the correct definition below. Some terms may not be used.

A. Cold chain

B. Conjugate vaccine

C. Live attenuated vaccine

D. Immunosuppressants

E. Immunization

F. Toxoid vaccine

G. Vaccine

H. Antigen

I. Immunomodulator

J. Inactivated, killed vaccine

1. A(n) _____ is a substance that prevents disease by taking advantage of your body's ability to make antibodies and release "killer" cells to disease.

2. The _____ is a set of safe handling practices that ensure vaccines and immunologic agents requiring refrigeration are maintained at a required temperature.

3. A(n) _____ links antigens or toxoids to polysaccharide or sugar molecules that certain bacteria use as a protective device to disguise themselves.

4. Drugs that inhibit cell proliferation are known as _____.

5. A vaccine that stimulates the immune system to produce antibodies to a specific toxin that causes illness is called a(n) _____.

6. A(n) _____ is a deliberate, artificial exposure to disease to produce acquired immunity.

7. _____ is a living but weakened version of a disease.

8. _____ is a chemical agent that modifies the immune response or the functioning of the immune system.

9. A substance, usually a protein fragment, that causes an immune response is a(n) _____.

10. _____ provides less immunity than live vaccines but has fewer risks for vaccine-induced disease.

MULTIPLE CHOICE

1. Inactivated, killed vaccine has _____ risk(s) for vaccine-induced disease.

   _____
   A. more
   B. little
   C. similar

2. Select the vaccine that is *not* recommended for children younger than 10 years. _____
   A. HepB
   B. DTP
   C. IPV
   D. HPV
   E. MMR

3. Select the **false** statement. Each time the cold chain is disrupted, _____.
   A. the effectiveness vaccine is reduced
   B. the loss of potency is cumulative
   C. the vaccine potency is unaffected
   D. the shelf life of the vaccine is reduced

4. Cold chain protocols for drugs should be established for all of the following *except* _____.
   A. receiving
   B. stocking
   C. storage
   D. transport
   E. administration

5. If the cold chain has been breached, pharmacy technicians should _____.
   A. notify the pharmacist
   B. isolate the drug(s) and label DO NOT USE
   C. discard the drug(s) if instructed
   D. document the breach
   E. all of the above

6. To maintain the cold chain, pharmacy technicians should _____.
   A. place drugs directly on ice-packs when shipping
   B. immediately stock vaccines in the refrigerator when required
   C. check refrigerator temperatures every 3 months
   D. place drugs requiring refrigeration near the freezer compartment

7. Whereas vaccines boost the immune response, immunopharmacologic drugs such as cyclosporine _____.
   A. suppress cells of the immune system
   B. boost cells of the immune system
   C. have no effect on cells of the immune system

8. Cyclosporine _____.
   A. is derived from a bacterium
   B. suppresses rejection of organ transplants
   C. suppresses interferon-α
   D. has product formulations that are substitutable

9. Select the drug that does *not* suppress or deplete T cells. _____
   A. cyclosporine
   B. antithymocyte globulin
   C. tacrolimus
   D. Enbrel

10. Which drug is administered for severe eczema?

    _____
    A. cyclosporine
    B. tacrolimus
    C. basiliximab
    D. daclizumab

FILL IN THE BLANK: DRUG NAMES

1. What is the **brand name** for Hib conjugate vaccine? _____

2. What is the **generic name** for Boostrix and Adacel? _____

3. What is the **generic name** for Havrix? _____

4. What is the **brand name** for meningococcal vaccine? _____

5. What is the **generic name** for Energix-B and Recombivax? _____

6. What is the **brand name** for pneumococcal polysaccharide 7-polyvalent vaccine?

   _____

7. What is the *generic name* for Varivax? _____

8. What is the *brand name* for pneumococcal polysaccharide 23-polyvalent vaccine?

   _____

9. What is the *generic name* for Rabavert? _____

10. What is the *generic name* for Sandimune and Neoral? _____

11. What is the *brand name* for sirolimus? _____

12. What is the *generic name* for Prograf and Protopic? _____

13. What is the *brand name* for muromonab-CD3? _____

14. What is the *generic name* for CellCept? _____

15. What is the *brand name* for basiliximab? _____

16. What is the *generic name* for Thymoglobulin? _____

17. What is the *brand name* for daclizumab? _____

18. What is the *generic name* for WinRho SDF and RhoGam? _____

19. What is the *brand name* for etanercept? _____

20. What is the *generic name* for Kineret? _____

MATCHING

Patient education is an essential component of therapeutics. Select the **best** warning label to apply to the prescription vial given to patients taking the drugs listed.

1. _____ Rh$_o$[D] immune globulin

2. _____ cyclosporine caps

3. _____ sirolimus

4. _____ Prograf

A. TAKE ON AN EMPTY STOMACH

B. REFRIGERATE; DISCARD WITHIN 30 DAYS OF OPENING

C. SWALLOW CAPSULES WHOLE; DON'T CRUSH OR CHEW

D. PROTECT FROM LIGHT

TRUE OR FALSE

1. _____ A live, attenuated vaccine can mutate to a virulent form of the disease.

2. _____ Cyclosporine oral liquids *nonmodified* (Sandimmune) is substitutable with cyclosporine oral liquid *modified* (Neoral, Gengraf).

3. _____ A common ending for monoclonal antibody immunomodulators is *-mab*.

4. _____ A common ending for macrolides used for immunosuppression is *-limus*.

5. _____ Rh$_o$[D] immune globulin is administered to pregnant women who are Rh (-) to prevent erythroblastosis fetalis.

CRITICAL THINKING

The following hard copy is brought to your pharmacy for filling. Identify the prescription error(s). (You already have the patient's full address on file.)

Anh Dang Tu, MD   Date _____
1145 Broadway
Anytown, USA
Pt. Name _____ Joan Neilsen _____
Address _____
℞   *Sandimune 100mg/ml*
15mg/kg in 2 divided doses daily
Refills _____
_____ *AD Tu* _____   _____
Substitution permitted   Dispense as written

1. Spot the error in the following prescription:

   _____

   A. Quantity missing
   B. Directions incomplete
   C. Strength missing
   D. Strength incorrect
   E. Dosage form incorrect

2. Give six pairs of drug names that have look-alike or sound-alike issues with drugs used to treat cancer.

DRUG NAME	LOOK-ALIKE OR SOUND-ALIKE DRUG

RESEARCH ACTIVITY

1. Pharmacists and pharmacy technicians play an important role in increasing community awareness of the importance of vaccination against vaccine preventable illnesses. Search the Internet, and identify community initiatives run by pharmacies to increase public awareness.

_____

_____

_____

_____

_____

39 Treatment of Fungal Infections

TERMS AND DEFINITIONS

Match each term with the correct definition below. Some terms may not be used.

A. Antifungal

B. *Candida*

C. Dermatophytes

D. Fungus (*pl.* fungi)

E. Mycoses

F. Onychomycosis

G. Ringworm

H. Vulvovaginal candidiasis

1. The general term for fungal infections is _____.

2. _____ are a group of fungi responsible for most fungal infections of the skin, hair, and nails.

3. _____ is a fungal infection involving the fingernails or toenails.

4. A drug used to treat a fungal infection is called a(n) _____.

5. Another name for _____ is yeast vaginitis.

6. A(n) _____ is an organism similar to plants but lacking chlorophyll and capable of producing mycotic (fungal) infections.

7. Although its common name is "yeast," _____ is a type of fungus.

8. _____ is a group of tinea infections involving the body or scalp.

MULTIPLE CHOICE

1. Select the method of reproduction that is *not* used by fungi. _____
   A. Budding
   B. Releasing spores
   C. Pollination
   D. Fusing hyphae (body of the fungus made of tiny filaments)

2. Which statement about ringworm is **false**?

   _____
   A. Infections are caused by a roundworm.
   B. Infections have a characteristic ringlike shape.
   C. Infections may be spread person to person.
   D. Infections may be spread animal to person.

3. Tinea capitis is a fungal infection located on the

   _____.
   A. torso
   B. fingernails
   C. scalp
   D. groin

4. A common ending for antifungal agents is

   _____.
   A. *-pramine*
   B. *-vir*
   C. *-mycin*
   D. *-azoles*

5. Select the drug that should *not* be taken concurrently

   with posaconazole. _____.
   A. sertraline
   B. nitroglycerin SL
   C. cimetidine
   D. sucralfate

6. Women may develop vaginal yeast infections when

   _____.
   A. the pH of the vagina becomes acidic
   B. they douche frequently
   C. drug therapy suppresses *Candida* growth
   D. they take broad spectrum antibiotics

7. Which recommendation will *not* decrease the risk
   for recurrent athlete's foot infections?

   _____
   A. Keep feet clean and dry.
   B. Avoid walking barefoot across the floor of public
      facilities.
   C. Wear nylon socks.
   D. Use antifungal powders.

8. Select the antifungal drug that can be obtained

   without a prescription. _____
   A. Diflucan
   B. Sporanox
   C. clotrimazole
   D. posaconazole

9. Clotrimazole is produced in all of the following

   dosage forms *except* _____.
   A. topical creams
   B. vaginal creams
   C. suppositories
   D. troche or lozenge
   E. capsule

10. Select the antifungal that is indicated for prevention

    of athlete's foot. _____
    A. tolnaftate
    B. nystatin
    C. terbinafine
    D. griseofulvin
    E. miconazole

FILL IN THE BLANK: DRUG NAMES

1. What is the *brand name* for fluconazole? _____

2. What is the *generic name* for Gynezole-1? _____

3. What is the *generic name* for Lotrimin (United States) and Canasten (Canada)? _____

4. What is the *brand name* for itraconazole? _____

5. What is the *generic name* for Spectazole (United States)? _____

6. What is the *brand name* for oxiconazole (United States)? _____

7. What is the *generic name* for Nizoral? _____

8. What is the *brand name* for voriconazole? _____

9. What is the *generic name* for Monistat? _____

10. What is a *brand name* for nystatin? _____

11. What is the *generic name* for Noxafil (United States) and Spriafil (Canada)? _____

12. What is the *brand name* for naftifine? _____

13. What is the *generic name* for Exelderm (United States)? _____

14. What is the *brand name* for tolnaftate? _____

15. What is the *generic name* for Terazole? _____

16. What is the *brand name* for caspofungin? _____

17. What is the *generic name* for Tioconastat (United States)? _____

18. What are *brand names* for ciclopirox? _____

19. What is the *generic name* for Mentax (United States)? _____

20. What is the *generic name* for Gris-PEG? _____

21. What is the *generic name* for Lamisil? _____

22. What is the *brand name* for undecylenic acid? _____

23. What is the *generic name* for Fungizone (Canada)? _____

24. What is the *generic name* for Natacyn? _____

25. What is the *generic name* for anidulafungin (United States)? _____

26. What is the *generic name* for Mycamine (United States)? _____

27. What is the *generic name* for Betadine? _____

MATCHING

Match the fungal infection to its location.

1. _____ mouth   A. tinea cruris

2. _____ scalp   B. tinea corporis

3. _____ groin   C. tinea unguium

4. _____ nails   D. thrush

5. _____ body   E. tinea capitis

TRUE OR FALSE

1. _____ Tinea unguium is also known as onychomycosis.

2. _____ Prescriptions written for griseofulvin ultramicrosize may be substituted with griseofulvin microsize.

3. _____ A common ending for echinocandin antifungals is *-fungin*.

4. _____ A common ending for allylamine antifungals is *-fungin*.

5. _____ Most fungal infections of the skin are caused by a group of fungi called dermatophytes.

6. _____ Women who take broad-spectrum antibiotics may develop a yeast infection.

7. _____ Products labeled for the treatment of jock itch should not be used to treat athlete's foot.

8. _____ Nystatin, natamycin, and amphotericin B are all derived for the fungi-like bacteria.

9. _____ Griseofulvin should be taken with a high fat content meal.

10. _____ *Candida* thrives in cool, dry areas.

CRITICAL THINKING

The following hard copies are brought to your pharmacy for filling. Identify the prescription error(s). (You already have the patient's full address on file.)

Anh Dang Tu, MD   Date _____
1145 Broadway
Anytown, USA

Pt. Name _____ Joan Neilson _____

Address _____

R̸ *Diflucan*

Take 2 tablets as a single dose   #2

Refills _____

_____ *AD Tu* _____

Substitution permitted   Dispense as written

---

1. Spot the error in the following prescription:

   _____

   A. Quantity missing
   B. Directions incomplete
   C. Strength missing
   D. Strength incorrect
   E. Dosage form incorrect

Anh Dang Tu, MD   Date _____
1145 Broadway
Anytown, USA

Pt. Name _____ Lili Ng _____

Address _____

R̸ *Noxafil 200mg/5ml*

   200mg TID   SHAKE WELL

Refills _____

_____ *AD Tu* _____

Substitution permitted   Dispense as written

---

2. Spot the error in the following prescription:

   _____

   A. Quantity missing
   B. Directions incorrect
   C. Strength missing
   D. Strength incorrect
   E. Dosage form incorrect

3. Give six pairs of drug names that have look-alike or sound-alike issues with drugs used to treat fungal infections.

DRUG NAME	LOOK-ALIKE OR SOUND-ALIKE DRUG

RESEARCH ACTIVITY

Access the Merck Manual Online's website (http://www.merck.com/mmpe/sec10/ch125/ch125c.html) and Family Doctor's website (http://familydoctor.org/online/famdocen/home/common/infections/common/fungal/663.printerview.html) to conduct research on onychomycosis.

1. What are risk factors for development of this condition?

_____

_____

_____

_____

_____

2. Why is onychomycosis so difficult to treat?

_____

_____

_____

_____

_____

40 Treatment of Decubitus Ulcers and Burns

TERMS AND DEFINITIONS

Match each term with the correct definition below. Some terms may not be used.

A. Blister

B. Decubitus ulcer

C. Eschar

D. Escharotomy

E. First-degree burn

F. Fourth-degree burn

G. Full-thickness burn

H. Partial-thickness burns

I. Second-degree burn

J. Third-degree burn

K. Debridement

L. Rule of nines

1. A(n) _____ involves underlying muscles, fasciae, or bone.

2. _____ is the process of removal of blackened and necrotic skin called _____.

3. A "bedsore" is a type of _____ or pressure sore.

4. A burn that involves deep epidermal layers and causes damage to the upper layers of dermis is called a(n) _____.

5. Injured area in which fluid collects below or within the epidermis as a result of a burn is called a(n) _____.

6. A(n) _____ causes minor discomfort and reddening of the skin.

7. A burn that is characterized by destruction of the epidermis and dermis is called a(n) _____.

8. First- and second-degree burns are also known as _____; in contrast, third-degree burns are known as _____.

9. _____ is a surgical removal of foreign material and dead tissue from a wound to prevent infection and promote healing.

10. _____ is a formula for estimating the percentage of adult body surface covered by burns dividing the body into 11 areas, each representing 9% of the body surface area.

MULTIPLE CHOICE

1. Which advice is *not* given to a person who has caught on fire? _____
   A. Stop
   B. Drop
   C. Roll
   D. Run

2. One formula for estimating the percentage of adult body surface covered by burns is called the _____.
   A. Rule of fives
   B. Rule of sevens
   C. Rule of nines
   D. Rule of 12s

3. A third-degree burn _____.
   A. involves deep epidermal layers and causes damage to the upper layers of dermis
   B. is characterized by destruction of the epidermis and dermis
   C. causes minor discomfort and reddening of the skin
   D. involves underlying muscles or bone

4. A decubitus ulcer may form from _____.
   A. prolonged pressure to an area
   B. continuous friction or rubbing against a surface
   C. prolonged exposure to cold
   D. all of the above

5. A stage IV wound is characterized by _____.
   A. surface reddening of the skin
   B. involvement of skin and underlying muscle, tendons, and bone
   C. blisters
   D. involvement through all layers of the skin

6. Debridement of dead tissue is accomplished by applying all of the following *except* _____.
   A. collagenase
   B. hydrocortisone
   C. papain and urea
   D. Granulex

7. The most commonly used topical medicine for the treatment of burns is _____.
   A. erythromycin ointment
   B. silver sulfadiazine cream
   C. butter
   D. hydrocortisone cream

8. Which of the following antiinfective drugs requires a prescription? _____
   A. bacitracin ointment
   B. triple antibiotic ointment
   C. Polysporin ointment
   D. Bactroban ointment

9. Select the wound care product that is used for antiseptic irrigation. _____
   A. aluminum acetate
   B. silver nitrate
   C. hydrocortisone

10. The most common adverse effect of mafenide is _____.
   A. itchiness
   B. burning
   C. coldness
   D. dry skin

FILL IN THE BLANK: DRUG NAMES

1. What is a **brand name** for bacitracin? _____

2. What is the **generic name** for Santyl? _____

3. What is the **generic name** for Accuzyme (United States)? _____

4. What is the **generic name** for Garamycin ointment? _____

5. What is the *generic name* for Granulex (United States)? _____

6. What is the *brand name* for mupirocin? _____

7. What is the *generic name* for Noritate cream? _____

8. What is the *generic name* for Silvadene (United States) and Flumazine (Canada)? _____

9. What is the *brand name* for mafenide? _____

10. What is the *generic name* for Betadine? _____

TRUE OR FALSE

1. _____ According to the rule of palms, a burn victim's palm size is equivalent to about 5% of total body surface area.

2. _____ There are three categories of burns (first, second, and third degree).

3. _____ An alternative name for first- and second-degree burns is partial-thickness burns.

4. _____ Air-permeable occlusive clear dressings promote healing of decubitus ulcers.

5. _____ Two common complications of burns are infection and edema.

CRITICAL THINKING

The following hard copies are brought to your pharmacy for filling. Identify the prescription error(s). (You already have the patient's full address on file.)

```
Anh Dang Tu, MD          Date _____
1145 Broadway
Anytown, USA

Pt. Name _____ Joan Neilson _____
Address _____
Rx   Silver sulfadiazine cream
        Apply once or twice daily with sterile-gloved hand


Refills _____
     ___ AD Tu ___          _____
Substitution permitted       Dispense as written
```

1. Spot the error in the following prescription:

    _____

    A. Quantity missing
    B. Directions incomplete
    C. Strength missing
    D. Strength incorrect
    E. Dosage form incorrect

```
Anh Dang Tu, MD          Date _____
1145 Broadway
Anytown, USA

Pt. Name _____ Lili Ng _____
Address _____
Rx   Santyl ointment    250 units/Gm
        apply once daily


Refills _____
     ___ AD Tu ___          _____
Substitution permitted       Dispense as written
```

2. Spot the error in the following prescription:

    _____

    A. Quantity missing
    B. Directions incorrect
    C. Strength missing
    D. Strength incorrect
    E. Dosage form incorrect

3. Give four pairs of drug names that have look-alike or sound-alike issues with drugs used to treat wounds.

DRUG NAME	LOOK-ALIKE OR SOUND-ALIKE DRUG

RESEARCH ACTIVITY

1. Some hospital pharmacies raise maggots. Conduct an Internet search to discover the current use of maggots in medicine and write a paragraph describing this process.

_____

_____

_____

_____

_____

_____

41 Treatment of Acne

TERMS AND DEFINITIONS

Match each term with the correct definition below. Some terms may not be used.

A. Acne

B. Blackhead

C. Comedones

D. Cysts

E. Keratolytic

F. Milia

G. Nodule

H. Papule

I. Pustule

J. Whitehead

K. Acne vulgaris

L. Desquamation

M. Pilosebaceous units (PSUs)

1. A(n) _____ agent is a peeling agent.

2. A(n) _____ is a large, inflamed lesion and may be superficial or deep.

3. _____ is a condition that results in the formation of _____, enlarged and plugged hair follicles.

4. A(n) _____ contains sebum and bacteria that have become trapped in the hair follicle and moves to the surface.

5. An obstructed follicle that becomes inflamed is called a(n) _____.

6. _____ are tiny little bumps that occur when normally sloughed skin cells get trapped in small pockets on the surface of the skin.

7. A pimple that contains trapped sebum and bacteria and stays below the skin surface is called a(n)

_____.

8. _____ is a ruptured pustule and can form an abscess.

9. The end products of pustules or nodules are called _____.

10. _____ is the most common form of acne.

11. _____ consists of a sebaceous gland connected to a canal, called a follicle, and contains a fine hair.

12. The shedding of the outer layers of the skin is known as _____.

MULTIPLE CHOICE

1. Factors that make acne worse include all of the following *except* _____.
   A. changing hormone levels in adolescence
   B. grease encountered in the work environment
   C. cosmetics
   D. chocolate
   E. stress

2. Drugs that can cause acne include all of the following

   except _____.
   A. lithium
   B. penicillin
   C. prednisone
   D. phenytoin

3. Blackheads turn black because of _____.
   A. melanin
   B. dirt
   C. bacteria
   D. hair

4. Acne is treated with administration of all of the

   following *except* _____.
   A. antibiotics
   B. keratolytics
   C. topical corticosteroids
   D. oral contraceptives

5. Women taking _____ must use birth control for at least 1 month before, during, and 1 month after a course of therapy.
   A. erythromycin
   B. isotretinoin
   C. benzoyl peroxide
   D. clindamycin

6. In the United States, prescribers, pharmacies, and patients are required to register in the FDA iPLEDGE

   program as a condition for use of _____ to minimize risks of birth defects.
   A. minocycline
   B. erythromycin
   C. isotretinoin
   D. tetracycline

7. Which topical medication is marketed for both prescription and nonprescription use?

   _____
   A. clindamycin gel
   B. erythromycin solution
   C. tazarotene
   D. benzoyl peroxide

8. _____ works by killing the bacteria that infect pores.
   A. Tazarotene
   B. Azelaic acid
   C. Adapalene
   D. Tretinoin

9. Which oral antiinfective is *not* a first-line treatment

   for acne? _____
   A. clarithromycin
   B. tetracycline
   C. erythromycin
   D. doxycycline
   E. minocycline

FILL IN THE BLANK: DRUG NAMES

1. What is the **brand name** for doxycycline? _____

2. What is the **generic name** for Panoxyl? _____

3. What is the **generic name** for SAStid? _____

4. What is the **brand name** for adapalene? _____

5. What is the **generic name** for Sulfacet-R? _____

6. What is the **generic name** for Azelex (United States) and Finacea (Canada)? _____

7. What is the **brand name** for benzoyl peroxide and erythromycin? _____

8. What is the **generic name** for A/T/S (United States) and Staticin? _____

9. What is the **brand name** for tazarotene? _____

10. What is the **generic name** for Benzaclin? _____

11. What is the **generic name** for Accutane? _____

12. What is the **generic name** for Minocin? _____

13. What is the **generic name** for Renova and Retin A? _____

14. What is the **generic name** for Ziana (United States)? _____

MATCHING

Patient education is an essential component of therapeutics. Select the **best** warning label to apply to the prescription vial given to patients taking the drugs listed.

1. _____ Retin A 0.025%

2. _____ tetracycline 500 mg

3. _____ benzoyl peroxide 10%

4. _____ erythromycin 250 mg delayed-release tab

5. _____ Accutane 20 mg

A. AVOID PREGNANCY

B. BLEACHING AGENT—AVOID CONTACT WITH FABRIC AND HAIR

C. AVOID PROLONGED SUNLIGHT; USE A SUNBLOCK; APPLY SPARINGLY

D. TAKE ON AN EMPTY STOMACH

E. TAKE WITH FOOD

TRUE OR FALSE

1. _____ Pilosebaceous units consist of a sebaceous gland connected to a hair follicle.

2. _____ A blackhead is a closed comedone.

3. _____ Acne vulgaris occurs most frequently in the adolescent years.

4. _____ Benzoyl peroxide may cause dry skin and redness.

5. _____ Acne outbreaks are typically more severe in girls than in boys.

6. _____ *Propionibacterium* is a bacterium that causes acne.

The following hard copies are brought to your pharmacy for filling. Identify the prescription error(s). (You already have the patient's full address on file.)

```
Anh Dang Tu, MD          Date _____
1145 Broadway
Anytown, USA

Pt. Name _____ John Neilson _____
Address _____

Rx    Retin-A gel    45Gm
      apply nightly


Refills _____
        AD Tu              _____
Substitution permitted      Dispense as written
```

1. Spot the error in the following prescription:

   _____

   A. Quantity missing
   B. Directions incomplete
   C. Strength missing
   D. Strength incorrect
   E. Dosage form incorrect

```
Anh Dang Tu, MD          Date _____
1145 Broadway
Anytown, USA

Pt. Name _____ Lili Newell _____
Address _____

Rx    Minocycline 100mg BID



Refills _____
        AD Tu              _____
Substitution permitted      Dispense as written
```

2. Spot the error in the following prescription:

   _____

   A. Quantity missing
   B. Directions incorrect
   C. Strength missing
   D. Strength incorrect
   E. Dosage form incorrect

3. Give six pairs of drug names that have look-alike or sound-alike issues with drugs used to treat acne.

DRUG NAME	LOOK-ALIKE OR SOUND-ALIKE DRUG

4. You are asked to compound clindamycin 2% solution from clindamycin 75-mg capsules and commercially prepared clindamycin 1% solution (60 mL). How many capsules will you need to add to the commercially prepared solution? Please show your calculations.

_____

_____

_____

_____

_____

RESEARCH ACTIVITY

1. Severe acne can be disfiguring. Access the National Library of Medicine's website (http://www.nlm.nih.gov/medlineplus/acne.html#cat11) and other websites to learn more about acne. Write a paragraph about the social impact of acne.

_____

_____

_____

_____

_____

42 Treatment of Eczema and Psoriasis

TERMS AND DEFINITIONS

Match each term with the correct definition below. Some terms may not be used.

A. Atopic

B. Atopic dermatitis

C. Cutaneous

D. Dermatitis

E. Eczema

F. Exacerbation

G. Phototherapy

H. Psoriasis

I. Remission

J. Plaque psoriasis

1. The term used to describe inflammation of the skin is _____.

2. _____ is a treatment for atopic dermatitis that involves exposing the skin to ultraviolet A or B light waves.

3. The term used to describe a group of diseases in which there is an inherited tendency to develop other allergic conditions is _____.

4. A chronic disease of the skin, _____ is characterized by itchy red patches covered with silvery scales.

5. _____ is a chronic allergic condition that affects the skin.

6. A general term used to describe several types of inflammation of the skin is _____.

7. _____ is the lessening in severity or an abatement of symptoms.

8. The aggravation of symptoms or increases in the severity of the disease is called _____.

9. _____ is a term that means pertaining to the skin.

10. _____ is the most common form of psoriasis.

MULTIPLE CHOICE

1. Irritants that aggravate the skin of persons with

   atopic dermatitis are _____.
   A. cotton and silk
   B. perfumes and cosmetics
   C. rice and potatoes
   D. cleaning solvents and detergents
   E. B and D

2. Psoriatic patches are typically found in all of the

   regions *except* _____.
   A. neck
   B. face
   C. elbows
   D. genitals
   E. hands and feet

3. Which advice would not be given to a person with

   eczema? _____
   A. Avoid wearing wool or clothing that feels
      "scratchy."
   B. Increase humidity in the household environment.
   C. Apply moisturizers and lotion to the skin.
   D. Take hot baths.

4. Of the following, the most potent corticosteroid

   classification is _____.
   A. class I
   B. class II
   C. class III
   D. class IV
   E. class V

5. Select the corticosteroid that is in the least potent

   category. _____
   A. clobetasol
   B. betamethasone dipropionate (optimized)
   C. hydrocortisone base cream
   D. halobetasol propionate
   E. fluocinonide

6. Which of the following adverse effects is not linked
   to topical use of corticosteroids?

   _____
   A. thinning of the skin
   B. Cushing syndrome
   C. stretch marks (striae)
   D. spider veins
   E. acne

7. Select the drug that is indicated for the treatment of

   severe psoriasis and arthritis. _____
   A. cyclosporine
   B. azathioprine
   C. methotrexate
   D. calcipotriene

8. Topical corticosteroids are used for the treatment of

   all of the following *except* _____.
   A. psoriasis
   B. seborrhea
   C. candidiasis
   D. eczema
   E. allergic dermatitis

9. The FDA and Health Canada require manufacturers
   to include a Black Box warning in the package

   insert for _____ describing the
   increased risks for cancer.
   A. Dermatop-E and Dovonex
   B. Cutivate and Ultravate
   C. methotrexate and Enbrel
   D. pimecrolimus and tacrolimus

10. Dovonex is a synthetic analog of

    _____.
    A. vitamin A
    B. vitamin B
    C. vitamin C
    D. vitamin D

FILL IN THE BLANK: DRUG NAMES

1. What is a **brand name** for betamethasone dipropionate? _____

2. What is the **generic name** for Aclovate (United States)? _____

3. What is the **generic name** for Luxiq (United States) and Valisone (Canada)? _____

4. What is the **brand name** for desoximetasone? _____

5. What is the **generic name** for Cyclocort (United States)? _____

6. What are **brand names** for fluocinolone acetonide? _____

7. What is the **generic name** for Clobex? _____

8. What is the **brand name** for fluticasone? _____

9. What is the **generic name** for Desowen (United States) and Desocort (Canada)? _____

10. What is the **brand name** for halcinonide? _____

11. What is the **generic name** for Nerisone (Canada)? _____

12. What is the **brand name** for halobetasol? _____

13. What is the **generic name** for Psorcon-E (United States)? _____

14. What is the **brand name** for hydrocortisone valerate? _____

15. What is the **generic name** for Lidex? _____

16. What is the **brand name** for prednicarbate? _____

17. What is the **generic name** for Hytone (United States) and Dermaflex HC (Canada)?

    _____

18. What is the **brand name** for pimecrolimus? _____

19. What is the **generic name** for Locoid (United States)? _____

20. What is the **brand name** for tacrolimus? _____

21. What is the **generic name** for Elocon (United States) and Elocom (Canada)? _____

22. What is the **brand name** for calcipotriene (United States) and calcipotriol (Canada)?

    _____

23. What is the **generic name** for Kenalog? _____

24. What is a **brand name** for methoxsalen? _____

25. What is the **generic name** for Taclonex (United States) and Dovobet (Canada)? _____

26. What is the **brand name** for azathioprine? _____

27. What is the **generic name** for Neoral? _____

28. What is the **brand name** for etanercept? _____

29. What is the **generic name** for Trexall? _____

30. What is the **generic name** for DrithoScalp and Psoriatec (United States)? _____

MATCHING

Match each drug to its pharmacological classification.

1. _____ Dovonex

2. _____ methotrexate

3. _____ mometasone

4. _____ Elidel

5. _____ Oxsoralen Ultra

A. furanocoumarins

B. corticosteroid

C. vitamin D analog

D. calcineurin inhibitor

E. immunosuppressants

MATCHING

Patient education is an essential component of therapeutics. Select the best warning label to apply to the prescription container given to patients taking the drugs listed.

1. _____ triamcinolone

2. _____ Oxsoralen Ultra

3. _____ cyclosporine

4. _____ Enbrel

5. _____ anthralin

A. AVOID PROLONGED EXPOSURE TO SUNLIGHT

B. APPLY SPARINGLY

C. REFRIGERATE; DO NOT FREEZE

D. SWALLOW WHOLE; DON'T CRUSH OR CHEW

E. MAY STAIN HAIR, CLOTHING, OR SKIN

TRUE OR FALSE

1. _____ Stress and dry skin may aggravate psoriasis.

2. _____ It is uncommon for eczema that has gone into remission in childhood to return with the onset of puberty.

3. _____ Corticosteroids are categorized into five potency categories.

4. _____ Topical corticosteroids possess antiinflammatory and immunosuppressive properties.

5. _____ Phototherapy involves exposing the skin to ultraviolet A, B, and C light waves.

6. _____ The vehicle (base) in which the corticosteroid is suspended has no influence on potency.

CRITICAL THINKING

The following hard copy is brought to your pharmacy for filling. Identify the prescription error(s). (You already have the patient's full address on file.)

```
+-----------------------------------------+
|        Anh Dang Tu, MD      Date _____  |
|         1145 Broadway                    |
|         Anytown, USA                     |
|                                          |
| Pt. Name _____ Joan Neilson _____  |
| Address _____  |
| Rx   triancinolone 0.025%    15Gm        |
|      apply sparingly to affected area TID|
|                                          |
|                                          |
| Refills _____                           |
|       AD Tu          _____   |
| Substitution permitted   Dispense as written |
+-----------------------------------------+
```

1. Spot the error in the following prescription:

   _____

   A. Quantity missing
   B. Directions incomplete
   C. Strength missing
   D. Strength incorrect
   E. Dosage form missing

2. Give six pairs of drug names that have look-alike or sound-alike issues with drugs used to treat eczema and psoriasis.

DRUG NAME	LOOK-ALIKE OR SOUND-ALIKE DRUG

RESEARCH ACTIVITY

1. Review Chapter 1 and research the Internet to learn about drug product formulation. Write a paragraph explaining why the potency of corticosteroids is influenced by the vehicle in which the drug is mixed.

   _____

   _____

   _____

   _____

   _____

43 Treatment of Lice and Scabies

TERMS AND DEFINITIONS

Match each term with the correct definition below. Some terms may not be used.

A. Lice

B. Nits

C. Nymph

D. Ovicidal

E. Parasite

F. Pediculicide

G. Scabies

H. Scabicide

1. An organism that benefits by living in, with, or on another organism is called a _____.

2. A(n) _____ is a drug that kills _____, a parasitic mite that causes infection.

3. A drug that is _____ is able to kill the eggs of lice.

4. Another name for head lice eggs is _____.

5. A drug that kills lice is called a(n) _____.

6. _____ are a group of parasites that can live on the body, scalp, or genital area of humans.

7. The term used to describe a baby louse is _____.

MULTIPLE CHOICE

1. Which parasite is *not* a louse? _____
   A. *Pediculus humanus capitis*
   B. scabies
   C. *Pediculus humanus corporis*
   D. *Phthirus pubis*

2. _____ is a parasitic infection classified as a sexually transmitted infection (STI).
   A. *Pediculus humanus capitis*
   B. scabies
   C. *Pediculus humanus corporis*
   D. *Phthirus pubis*

3. Pharmacy technicians should apply the warning label

   _____ to prescription vials containing lindane shampoo.
   A. SHAKE WELL
   B. DILUTE BEFORE USE
   C. FOR EXTERNAL USE ONLY
   D. APPLY SPARINGLY

4. Which warning should be given to persons receiving a prescription for malathion? _____
   A. AVOID OPEN FLAMES (e.g., LIT CIGARETTES, CIGARS, AND PIPES)
   B. MAY STAIN CLOTHING AND HAIR
   C. MAY BLEACH CLOTHING AND HAIR
   D. DILUTE BEFORE USE

5. Select the drug for which the FDA requires manufacturers to place a Black Box warning in the package insert. _____
   A. lindane
   B. permithrins
   C. pyrethrins
   D. crotamiton

6. Select the drug that is contraindicated in infants. _____
   A. crotamiton
   B. lindane
   C. permethrins
   D. pyrethrins

7. Permethrin lotion should remain on the body for at least _____ hours before washing off.
   A. 2
   B. 4
   C. 6
   D. 8

8. Which of the following statements about body lice is **false**? _____
   A. Body lice infestations are caused by the parasite *Pediculus humanus corporis*.
   B. Adult body lice can survive away from a human host for 30 days.
   C. Body lice infestations are a serious public health concern.
   D. Body lice may cause epidemics of typhus and louse-borne relapsing fever.

9. In which environmental conditions does scabies thrive? _____
   A. dense populations such as in prisons and nursing homes
   B. warm environment
   C. moist environment
   D. arid environment
   E. scarcely populated environment

10. Strategies to prevent lice reinfestation include all of the following *except* _____.
   A. Treat all household members.
   B. Wash clothing, linens, and bedding in hot water.
   C. Throw away toys, clothing, and bedding that cannot be washed.
   D. Use a nit comb to remove eggs.

FILL IN THE BLANK: DRUG NAMES

1. What is the *generic name* for Ovide (United States)? _____

2. What is the *brand name* for crotamiton? _____

3. What is the *generic name* for Elimite (United States) and NIX? _____

4. What is the *generic name* for RID (United States) and R&C (Canada)? _____

TRUE OR FALSE

1. _____ Treatment of head lice requires shaving the head.

2. _____ Malathion was withdrawn from the market in Canada but is still available in the United States.

3. _____ Head lice most commonly affects children ages 3 to 11 years.

4. _____ Head lice infestation is caused by poor hygiene.

5. _____ Individuals *cannot* get pubic lice from sitting on public toilet seats.

6. _____ Permethrin is approved for the treatment of head lice, body lice, and pubic lice.

7. _____ Permethrin is ovicidal (kills eggs), but pyrethrins are not.

8. _____ Systemic absorption of lindane only occurs through broken skin.

9. _____ Permethrins and pyrethrins may only be obtained by prescription.

CRITICAL THINKING

The following hard copy is brought to your pharmacy for filling. Identify the prescription error(s). (You already have the patient's full address on file.)

| Anh Dang Tu, MD   Date _____ |
| 1145 Broadway |
| Anytown, USA |

Pt. Name _____ Julie Nelson _____

Address _____

℞ crotamiton 10% cream
Apply after bathing to the skin over the entire body from the chin to the toes. Repeat in 24 hours. Bathe 48 hours AFTER second dose.

Refills _____

_____ AD Tu _____   _____

Substitution permitted   Dispense as written

1. Spot the error in the following prescription:

   _____

   A. Quantity missing
   B. Directions incomplete
   C. Strength missing
   D. Strength incorrect
   E. Dosage form missing

2. Give one pair of drug names that have look-alike or sound-alike issues with drugs used to treat lice and scabies.

DRUG NAME	LOOK-ALIKE OR SOUND-ALIKE DRUG

RESEARCH ACTIVITY

1. Conduct an Internet search on the use of antiparasitic agents and antibiotics in agriculture. Write a paragraph explaining how their use may affect the treatment of infection in humans.

   _____

   _____

   _____

   _____

   _____